For Jacqui

Acknowledgements

In undertaking to prepare a study of an issue as multifaceted and as rapidly evolving as drug abuse in sport I have accumulated a number of debts which I am happy to have the opportunity to acknowledge. Particular thanks are due to George Walker, Head of the Sports Section of the Council of Europe, whose encyclopaedic knowledge of sport and extensive contacts throughout Europe and beyond were invaluable. Thanks are also due to Suzanne Little and Dominique Huber, also of the Sports Section, who dealt with my frequent requests for documents with great patience and good humour. Dr Michael Turner read through Chapter 3 and helped me clarify my analysis and avoid a number of errors. Michele Verroken of the United Kingdom's Sports Council's Ethics and Anti-doping Directorate read through the draft and provided important advice that enabled me to sharpen my argument. The opinions expressed in the book are, of course, my own as is the responsibility for any errors that remain.

Finally, thanks are due to Barbara Zatlokal of Council of Europe Publishing for her support and gentle encouragement to keep to deadlines.

Barrie Houlihan
Loughborough University

Contents

Preface 9

Chapters

1 The value of sport 11

2 The evolution of doping 33

3 Banned substances and practices and their effects 57

4 Beyond sport: doping and anti-doping policy 85

5 Defining the problem: the ethics of doping 107

6 The evolution of anti-doping policy: problems and solutions 129

7 Policy harmonisation: problems and prospects 153

8 The future of anti-doping policy 171

Appendices

A International Olympic Committee list of prohibited classes of substances and prohibited methods 191

B Anti-doping Convention, 1989 199

C State of ratification of signatures 209

Preface

The world of sport has long been blighted by the problem of drug use and misuse. Why is it that the strategies used to address the key issues are seemingly ineffective? Essential to any understanding of this question is an analysis of the key players, their interest in, and contribution to, progress towards drug free sport.

Barrie Houlihan has taken a critical look at this vital issue, particularly at the power relationships between key stakeholders and the fortunes of the athletes involved. The first chapter describes how the evolution of doping is intrinsically linked to sports policy development. Doping does not occur in isolation from other factors. For those who are keen to study the area in more depth, the examination of policy and, at times, contradictory practice can be found here. Yet the book goes further, by seeking out possible explanations and motivations.

Sport has not yet faced up to the vexing question of whether the issue is one of performance enhancement or the health of the athlete. Is it abuse or simply the detection of poorly defined substances? Certainly popular press headlines expose the irony of a situation where an athlete's performance is more important than life itself. Chapter 2 takes an historical look at the various substances, and the social and sporting context of misuse that has identified them as not quite the scientific achievements of which society should be proud.

Definitions should be the cornerstone of policy, and yet the guardians of sports ethics – both governments and sports organisations – have found this a major challenge to their credibility on the whole issue. Chapter 3 examines the link between awareness of misuse in sport and perceived ergogenic value, revealing the nature of misuse to be more sport-specific.

Houlihan argues that if competitive sport is justified in seeking greater advantage by the misuse of drugs – external rewards being a key motivation – how does one explain the increasing use of enhancing substances in the culture of recreational sport? Attitudes towards drug use in recreational sport represent one end of the continuum of sporting activity while at the opposite end the expectations upon elite athletes are entirely different. The lack of consensus in the sports world is explored in Chapter 4 as part of the problem sport itself has in addressing drug misuse. Demand reduction and sports testing programmes appear to be worlds apart, further complicated by apparent policy ambiguities among the sports organisations themselves. Anti-drugs strategies have taken many forms – in principle carrot and stick – but with varying degrees of impact. Perhaps the most alarming issue to emerge is the absence of success, if that is measured by the eradication of the problem.

Defining doping in respect of sporting ethics is shown as entirely plausible but seems unable to unite the sports world. Hence the apparent ambivalence that sports organisations seem to show to the «amateur» athlete and any argument of fairness. The sporting community and the business of sport are not easy to unite, as Chapter 5 shows us.

The recent history of anti-doping policy is the main focus of Chapter 6. A plethora of organisations, seemingly facing in the same direction but achieving different things, is provocatively examined. The political relationship between sport and government is probably at its most fascinating when considering the development of anti-doping policy. An understanding of the complexity of the issue and a certain dynamism, Houlihan points out, are important to the assessment of progress. Progress has been made, as Chapter 6 clearly shows: this has not always occurred without direct government intervention, but doping is now at the top of the sporting agenda.

Policy harmonisation is, in principle, the key to resolution of the problems that beset the anti-doping movement. It recognises the globalisation of sporting competition and is supportive of the fairness of sports participation. Regrettably, as Chapter 7 explains, it begs the question of whose standards are to be adopted – those of the highest or lowest denominator – as well as roles and responsibilities that are contentious. Among all the harmonisation efforts, those of the Council of Europe have perhaps made the greatest impact over the largest geographical, sporting and political area. The Council of Europe's Anti-doping Convention encompasses legislation as well as setting out strategies for compliance based on financial support. Government support for the infrastructure necessary to achieve the high standards required to give confidence to athletes, and to reduce the number of successful legal challenges, is closely monitored by the convention, although the next step towards international legislation may not be so far away.

And what of the future? In Chapter 8, Houlihan identifies the concern that must surely be felt by athletes over the apparent slowing of progress, the obstacles that seem to be insurmountable, or at least the absence of co-ordinated efforts to address them. Will there be a loss of interest in the fight against doping? Is it too confusing? Has it become too technical, needing resolution by super-scientists? Replacing anti-doping efforts with an all-pervading cynicism would sound the death-knell of sport. No responsible parent would put their child in the hands of sports coaches and medical people with ethical values based on the cynical misuse of drugs. If they are not good enough without drugs, maybe they are just not good enough. After all, it is only a game!

Michele Verroken
Director, Ethics and Anti-doping
United Kingdom Sports Council

Chapter 1

The value of sport

His tomb is thronged about at the altar where many strangers pass;
   but the glory
of Pelops flashes afar from Olympia
in the courses where speed is matched with speed
and a man's force harsh at the height.
And the winner the rest of his lifetime
keeps happiness beside him sweeter than honey

as far as the games go; but the day to day excellence
is best that can come to any man.

Pindar[1]

The quadrennial Olympic Games epitomise modern sport. The six or seven years of planning by the host city, the hundreds of television companies that broadcast the games, the thousands of participants, coaches, and officials that attend, and the hundreds of millions who watch the events from all points of the globe provide ample testimony to the prestige, popularity and global coverage of modern international sport. But it is not just the scale of the Olympic Games that sticks in the mind. The Olympics also provide an insight into the hold that sport has on the popular imagination. To reflect on the most memorable events of the last two or three games provides a rich range of images of triumph and despair, unanticipated success and unexpected failure, and breathtaking good fortune and heartbreaking bad luck.

This range of images and emotions could be found in any major international sports competition such as the Soccer World Cup, the Tour de France, and the World Athletics Championships. More importantly these images and emotions can also be found, and for many of us experienced, in the vast array of sport played by those whose sporting aspirations are far more modest. Yet sports participation provides a powerful thread that links the Olympic gold medalists, Stephen Redgrave and Matthew Pinsent, and the Saturday afternoon rowers, Sonia O'Sullivan, Haile Gabresilasie, and Moses Kiptanui and fun-runners in the Berlin marathon, and Jurgen Klinsman and Renaldo

---

1. Odes of Pindar, trans. R. Lattimore, 2nd edition, Chicago, University of Chicago Press, 1976.

and the thousands playing in the Sunday morning soccer leagues. In addition to the many millions throughout the world who participate in sport there is also the enormous number who experience the excitement of sport vicariously through spectating either at live events or through the media, especially television.

The extensiveness and intensity of popular involvement in sport and its capacity to arouse an astonishing depth of passion both in participants and spectators is only part of the reason for sport's unique place in modern society. The particularity of sport in the modern world is also based on the fact that sport is a cornerstone of the global corporate media provision and is the subject of intense government interest. In addition, modern sport is also remarkable for the degree to which it stirs, on the one hand, associations with a classical past, and on the other a belief that sport occupies a privileged position in society.

The deliberate association of sport with a classical past, especially through the Olympic Games, continues to provide a rich basis for the assumption of continuity with what many consider to be a time when sport was practised in a purer form and was less tarnished by its current association with excessive commercialism, professionalism, violence and drug abuse. For the founder of the modern Olympics, Pierre de Coubertin, the ancient Olympic Games provided a profound and powerful source of inspiration. The description of ancient games found in Homer' s poems, the *Iliad* and the *Odyssey*, provide a sharp insight into the interweaving of the athletic achievements of the warrior elite with the celebration of sport as an integral part of Hellenic culture. More importantly, Homer also makes clear the extent to which games and sports reflected a cultural ideal based on the complementarity of physical and intellectual excellence. The emphasis on the development of mind and body was based on a belief that true excellence was the product not just of physical prowess but of moral and intellectual qualities as well and provided "a profoundly original conception and a philosophy of life" that still resonates in our modern world and is particularly clearly reflected in the Olympic Charter.[1] As McIntosh notes, "[that] sport in the days of Homeric heroes was noble there is no doubt", but he also draws attention to the fact that in later years "the religious and cultural functions of the Olympic Games and of other Panhellenic festivals were obscured and then destroyed by specialism and commercialism" and that "success in the games was sought for narrow political ends both by states and by individuals".[2]

The desire to maintain continuity between ancient and modern sport, albeit based on a selective reading of the history of the ancient games, in part

1. Segrave, J.O & Chu, D. (eds.), *The Olympic Games in Transition*, Human Kinetics Books, Champaign, Illinois, 1988.
2. McIntosh, P., *Sport in Society*, (revised ed.), London, West London Press, 1987, pp. 20, 22 and 23.

explains the strong tendency to see modern sport as either outside normal society or at least as occupying a privileged position in society. At one extreme, sport is seen as providing an oasis within the modern world where higher standards of morality, often the product of a romanticisation of late Victorian middle class values, are practised as compared to the dubious and compromised character of everyday social, political and business behaviour. In part this view is based on a belief that it is possible to sustain values within sport that are not simply a reflection of those that are to be found in wider society, and thus expressions such as "fair play" and that "participating is more important than winning" are much used in competitive sport. Some substance is given to this assertion by emphasising the central place in sport of rules and their strict application. Much of modern sport is organised on a strictly meritocratic basis where quantification not only ensures that he or she who jumps higher, runs faster or throws further wins but also provides part of a clear and transparent set of rules of competition that, far from producing athletes that are "indoctrinated, regimented and repressed", provide liberation from prejudice and bias.[1]

If aspiration to a higher morality is part of the explanation for the distinctive position of sport in modern society, then an equally powerful contribution is made by the long association between amateurism and sporting excellence. In most European and North American countries the commitment to amateurism that dominated the bulk of the present century has left an indelible imprint on contemporary sport. For many, the legitimacy of sport's claim to higher moral values was reinforced by a definition of amateurism that attempted to protect competitive sport, and especially Olympic sport, from the corruption that prize money was thought to create.

Unfortunately, these views of modern and ancient sport are both highly inaccurate. Being generous, one might argue that to see modern sport as characterised by simple straightforward values which provide a model for wider society is not only to read selectively the history of ancient Greece, but also to romanticise the motives for the defence of amateurism in the nineteenth and twentieth centuries. A harsher but more accurate explanation is that the promoters of modern Olympic sport sought in the history of the early Olympics a rationale which would legitimise their preferred model of athletics which was designed to maintain the social position and interests of a privileged leisured class. It is indisputable that the pattern of sport that develops in a society is the product of that society in exactly the same way as the commercial and political systems are the product of deeper social values and attitudes. However, the suggestion that sport is as much the product of society as business and politics is not to detract from the desire that many involved in sport have to aspire to a set of values frequently less visible in other sectors of society. If sport has a contribution to make to the moral development of

1. Brohm, J.-M., *Sport, A Prison of Measured Time*, London, Pluto Press, (1978), p. 112.

society, it is in the persistence of an optimistic view of human nature and a belief that sport and major sports events are capable of demonstrating the viability of higher moral standards in modern complex societies. There is no better example of the seriousness of the challenge facing sport than the protracted campaign to eradicate doping from competitive sport. The anti-doping campaign can be seen as an acid test for the moral aspirations of national and international organisations involved in sport. Needless to say, the existence and strength of these aspirations must be explored through an analysis of the evidence rather than relying simply on assertion.

The recent Olympic Games in Atlanta provide an ideal starting point for an exploration of the place of sport in the contemporary world. The 1996 Olympic Games at Atlanta produced some magnificent sporting performances and also one of the lowest totals for positive drug tests at a recent games. Taken at face value the small number of doping positives was a major cause for optimism that the fight against cheating is being won. Yet such a view would be misleading, as a focus solely on the total number of positive test results would be to ignore a number of worrying incidents that indicate the depth and variability of the drugs problem in modern sport. Take first the fate of two Irish athletes, Michelle Smith and Marie McMahon. Smith, who lives and trains in Holland, stunned the Atlanta games by unexpectedly winning three gold and one bronze medals in the Olympic pool. Despite congratulations from President Clinton (conscious of the importance of the Irish-American vote for his chances of success in the forthcoming Presidential election) and being met on her return to Ireland by the Irish President (also aware of a good photo-opportunity), she was subject to a sustained campaign of innuendo and rumour suggesting that her success was due to drugs. That she had tested negative for drugs on many previous occasions was ignored and much was made of the facts that her improvement had been dramatic, and that her trainer and husband, Erik de Bruin, had tested positive in 1993 and was subsequently banned for four years. Marie McMahon had a less successful games failing to qualify for the 5000 metres finals. However, she did make headlines by failing a drug test which showed traces of phenylpropanolamine. In escaping a ban, the International Olympic Committee (IOC) commented that not only was she foolish for not having consulted a doctor before taking tablets to counter influenza symptoms but that she had not been properly advised about banned substances.

Both these episodes highlight difficulties in implementing an anti-doping strategy. The first difficulty is illustrated by Michelle Smith who is typical of the modern athlete, who will travel the world not only to compete but also to train, and as such draws attention to the need for an anti-doping strategy which is international rather than focused on the individual nation. But both Smith and McMahon also illustrate the need to have anti-doping strategies, which embrace education as well as testing, clearly in place in all countries. At the time when serious allegations were souring the pleasure of unaccustomed Olympic success, Ireland was unable to point to an existing policy for combating drug abuse among Irish athletes. In McMahon's case the absence of an anti-doping policy with a clear objective to educate and inform about drugs contributed to the embarrassment experienced by athletes. The fact that Smith (now Michelle de Bruin) was banned for four years in 1998 by the international swimming federation, FINA, for attempting to manipulate a test only added to the embarrassment that the domestic federation and the government experienced in the weeks after the Atlanta games.[1]

The second episode from the Atlanta games is a much more serious cause for concern and relates to the behaviour of four Russian athletes. Since the collapse of communism central and eastern European countries have been faced with an uphill struggle to live down their reputation for relying on state-sanctioned doping for much of their dominance of many post-war Olympic Games. For the former German Democratic Republic and the former Soviet Union the evidence was especially damning. At Atlanta four Russian athletes, a sprinter, two swimmers and a wrestler, tested positive for bromantan, a substance apparently developed to help Soviet soldiers stay alert during the Afghan war and which acts not only as a stimulant, but which may also be used as a masking agent for other drugs. The initial response of the IOC was to strip the wrestler Zafar Guliyev of his bronze medal and to indicate that a similar decision would be made regarding the bronze medal-winning swimmer, Andrei Korneyev. However, in their appeal to the Court of Arbitration for Sport, the Russians did not deny drug use, nor allege errors in the laboratory analysis, nor indeed rely on any of the other standard defences employed by those testing positive: the Russians simply argued that bromantan was not a banned substance. The argument of the Russian team was successful: the IOC decision was overturned and the two bronze medals were reinstated. Although the IOC considered the drug to be a stimulant and a masking agent, the committee's position was undermined because it had not, at the time of the Atlanta games, been added to the list of proscribed substances. In February 1997, bromantan was added to the IOC list of banned substances and practices but unfortunately too late for the two athletes who were denied a bronze medal in the wrestling and in swimming events by bromantan-using Russian athletes. What is particularly serious about this episode is what it reveals about the attitude of athletes and officials to the spirit of the IOC anti-doping policy. The IOC rules on doping appear to have been perceived as an impediment to success rather than as a reflection of Olympic values.

The third episode from Atlanta concerns the doubts expressed by the respected American scientist Don Catlin, who, for many years, has been at

---

1. Michelle de Bruin has denied that she attempted to manipulate the drug test by mixing whiskey with her urine sample to mask the presence of drugs and is currently appealing against the four year ban.

15

the forefront of research into methods to combat and detect drug abuse. In November 1996 Dr Catlin, who was in charge of the testing procedure for steroids at the Atlanta games, revealed that four positive results had not been released. According to the IOC, the problem lay in the sophistication of the much vaunted high-resolution mass spectrometer which, in the pre-games publicity, was claimed to posses the sensitivity to detect much lower levels of steroids in a urine sample. Unfortunately, it was the very sensitivity and sophistication of the equipment that led the IOC to discount the four positive results. The four positives were apparently based on the identification of such very low levels of steroids that the IOC medical commission was "not convinced that such traces of steroids constitute[d] doping".[1] Catlin's concerns were reinforced by the Penn State University epidemiologist, Chuck Yesalis, who accused the IOC of not spending enough money on anti-doping research which would enable a confident interpretation of test results. The failure to act on the 1996 positive results is not the first time that the IOC has been accused of inaction. During the 1984 Olympics, also held in the United States, nine positive results were treated in the same way although on this occasion the head of the IOC medical commission claimed that the confidential documents that enable the anonymous coded test results to be identified had inadvertently been shredded.

In addition to a concern at the failure of the IOC to act on the 1996 positives, Dr. Catlin also expressed his unease at the use of a private company, Smith-Kline, to undertake the testing of samples on the grounds that the firm, as one of the world's major pharmaceutical manufacturers, might be subject to a conflict of interest. "I don't think it's fair. SmithKline make testosterone, which is a very effective anabolic agent. They also make testosterone patches, which administer the steroid through the skin. I wish these products just weren't on the market," he is quoted as saying.[2] Among the issues raised by the actions of the IOC at both the 1984 and the 1996 Olympic Games are the increasing costs of keeping ahead of drug users, the increasing sophistication of the drugs being taken, and consequently the rising cost of developing, purchasing and operating the equipment and techniques required to monitor drug use. Related questions concern who should be expected to pay for testing and, more importantly, for the research effort necessary to keep abreast of changes in doping practices.

The final episode from the Atlanta games concerns the decision to allow two athletes to compete despite the fact that they both tested positive for drugs prior to the games. In May 1996 the Australian sprinter, Dean Capobianco, tested positive for steroids at a meeting in Holland. No action was taken against him because an Australian tribunal cleared him of any doping infraction, citing possible flaws in the drug-testing procedures. The international

1. The *Guardian* newspaper (UK), 28.11.1996.
2. The *Observer* newspaper (UK), 17.11.1996.

federation for track and field, The International Amateur Athletic Federation (IAAF), challenged the Australian decision and decided to take the case to an international arbitration panel, but as the panel was unable to be convened before the Olympic Games, Capobianco was allowed to compete. Similar circumstances surrounded the participation of the Italian high jumper, Antonella Bevilacqua, who tested positive twice in May 1996 for the banned drug ephedrine but was supported in her appeal by her domestic governing body who accepted her defence that she had taken the substance unwittingly in a Chinese herbal preparation. The IAAF considered the case against the athlete to be watertight and expected to win the case when it was considered by the federation's arbitration tribunal. However, fearing a legal challenge she was also permitted to participate in the Atlanta games. The decision of the federation is not in question but what the Capobianco and Bevilacqua cases exemplify is the trend within anti-doping policy towards an ever-increasing involvement of lawyers, the courts and arbitration panels at both the domestic and international levels with all the attendant problems of cost and complexity. Also, and more importantly, these cases draw attention to the need for due process to be observed in dealing with allegations of doping so as to protect the interests of both the athlete and the federation, and in addition draw attention to the need for close co-operation between the international federations and the domestic governing bodies if an anti-doping policy is to be successful.

The complexity surrounding the issue of doping is not just confined to the Olympic Games. More recently the 1998 Tour de France was disrupted by a series of doping allegations involving the use of erythropoietin (EPO), a drug which is claimed to be of benefit in endurance events. The main investigation is focused on Lille where the Festina team vehicle was searched and found to be carrying drugs. However, police investigations were, in autumn 1998, underway in eleven locations in France. Police searched the houses of team trainers in Italy and similar investigations were conducted in Belgium involving the staff and riders associated with the Festina and Lotto teams. Although investigations are still in progress, over fifty cyclists and support personnel have been interviewed by French police and thirteen have been charged. The incidents surrounding the 1998 Tour were remarkable not just because of the investigation which at one time threatened to bring the event to a premature end, but because of the scale of involvement of the French public authorities. In 1989 France passed a law which made it a criminal offence to supply certain drugs at sports events. Although much of the current publicity concerns the abusers of EPO, the focus of the police investigation is on those who supplied the cyclists. However, the involvement of the police and investigating magistrate has marginalised the domestic federation which suspended its own investigations pending completion of the public investigations.

While the continuing investigations of the 1998 Tour de France may prove to be significant for the future of the event and professional cycling, the four episodes from the last Olympic Games, taken individually, are neither especially dramatic nor unusual. Broadly similar disputes and issues could be selected from any recent Olympic Games or indeed from many other major international sports competitions. However, they do help to illustrate the modern context for high performance sport which can be characterised as an intensely commercialised and professionalised activity, in which governments and public authorities are taking an ever-increasing interest and where winning rather than taking part is considered by many athletes to be the only priority. In addition, there is a significant proportion of athletes who are willing to cheat in order to win or remain competitive at the elite level.

To treat these characteristics of modern sport as representing in some way a fall from grace would be to grossly over-romanticise the past. As will be shown, doping has a long history. The intention in the sections that follow is to identify the major elements of the social, economic and political context within which sport, doping and doping control takes place. It is only through an understanding of the context of modern sport that an appreciation of the problems facing those concerned with the effective development and implementation of anti-doping policy can be achieved.

Sport, government and nationalism

There is a temptation to equate governmental intervention in sport for political purposes with the period of the cold war. It is also common in the west to suggest that government manipulation of sport was a phenomenon found in the countries of the former communist bloc. Not only are both these assertions false but they also mislead in suggesting that government involvement in sport is a recent phenomenon. Indeed, it is likely that government involvement in sport is as old as organised sport itself. A review of the ancient Olympics states that there was "hardly a limit to the ways in which the passion for athletics and for victories could be capitalised on for ends that were in a broad sense political".[1] One of the examples given is the desire of rulers to enhance their status through association with successful athletes, a desire which led, on occasion, to attempts to "buy" or "transfer" elite athletes. Other examples include the recruitment of elite athletes as ambassadors and the use of athletic achievement in the Olympics to provide the foundation for a future political career. The close involvement of the Spanish royal family in the Barcelona Olympic Games, the visit to Wembley stadium by Helmut Kohl for one of Germany's matches in the Euro '96 soccer competition, and the journey by Charles Haughey, the Irish Prime Minister, to Paris to be there to welcome Stephen Roche as he crossed the finish line to win the 1987 Tour de France, all testify to the persistence of the original Greek belief that association with successful athletes enhances political status and popularity. The decision by the British Government to send Roger Bannister on a tour of the

---

1. Finley, M.I. & Pleket, H.W., *The Olympic Games, The First Thousand Years*, London, Chatto & Windus (1976).

United States following his sub-four-minute mile is one of many post-war examples of the use of successful athletes as ambassadors.

For many governments, apart from occasional interventions to regulate sport, their most consistent involvement has been through support for school sport. However, few governments until very recently saw school sport as part of a broader sport strategy: for most governments school sport was defined by its relationship to an education agenda which justified the inclusion of sport and physical education in the curriculum in terms of the beneficial impact on discipline and "character" on the one hand or health and hygiene on the other. It is only comparatively recently that governments have incorporated the funding of sport and recreation within a broadening conception of the role of the state, a conception that has extended beyond the regulation of sport to an acceptance of sport (and recreation) as an important part of the quality of life of developed societies.

For many developed industrial countries, even those such as the United States with a tradition of limited government, the provision of sport and recreation services by government has become gradually accepted. Almost uniformly across Europe and north America, local government has expanded the provision of sports facilities and increasingly the provision of staff, acknowledging that sport and recreation are important elements in the range of local services. For most countries the expansion of state involvement in sport and recreation services has been the result of a steadily widening conception of the role of the state to embrace a general responsibility for the quality of life and a much more broadly defined notion of welfare. Within democratic states the interplay between political parties and sports interest groups has also been supported by the attractiveness to the electorate of high-quality sport and recreation facilities.

In some countries the steady expansion of local provision has frequently taken place with the permission of central government rather than as a result of its explicit encouragement. However, for a number of other countries central government has frequently intervened to shape local provision where it defines sport as a useful policy instrument to solve specific social, economic or political problems. In many countries in western Europe, sport has been used as a palliative for a series of social problems including unemployment, juvenile delinquency and community fragmentation. In the United Kingdom, for example, sport has been seen as one of the solutions to the "problem of leisure" caused by the emergence of a generation of young males in the early post-war period who, by comparison to earlier generations, enjoyed relatively high wages and relatively short working hours which provided a substantial amount of free time.

The most notable change in the relationship between government and sport over the last fifty years has been the shift away from occasional involvement by the former in sport, to a situation where governments are now an integral part of the sports infrastructure in almost all countries in Europe and throughout the world. Indeed, until the early 1960s sport was of only marginal interest to most governments prompting sporadic, though occasionally forceful, interventions in reaction to specific problems such as urban disorder, poor standards of health in urban areas, or military requirements. Intervention by government was rarely the consequence of the recognition of sport and recreation as a distinct policy area. Nevertheless, in most countries there is a series of recurring themes that provide a significant degree of continuity and similarity in the pace and character of government involvement in the policy area.

One theme concerns the intervention by government to control aspects of sport such as hunting, bare-knuckle-fighting and bear-baiting, or to control activities associated with sport, particularly gambling. Legislative intervention was often designed to preserve class privileges and property rights under the guise of humanitarianism. In seventeenth-century England, the game laws were used to restrict access to particular field sports such as hunting. Similar laws existed in France, up until the revolution, which reserved all forms of game hunting, with the exception of rabbits, for the nobility.[1] More recently, in 1835 Britain passed the Cruelty to Animals Act which clearly reflected the exercise of power to preserve aristocratic and middle class privilege outlawing bull- and bear-baiting, which were both predominantly urban working class "sports", but leaving fox and stag hunting unrestricted. Similar examples could be drawn from the history of disputes over access to the countryside.[2]

A second theme in the development of sports policy is a sporadic concern with the health benefits of recreation and sport. In the nineteenth century the stimulus for concern was the appalling conditions in the rapidly expanding industrial towns and cities. Most countries in Europe passed public health legislation that helped to lay the basis of an urban infrastructure for sport. The Baths and Wash-houses Act, which was passed by the United Kingdom Parliament in 1846, gave powers to local authorities to build facilities to improve the standards of personal hygiene of the urban poor. Later, in 1936, the Public Health Act gave explicit recognition to the recreational role of public baths by enabling local authorities to build baths exclusively designed for swimming. A similar pattern of the adaptation of public health legislation for sport and recreational purposes can be traced through the history of the development of urban open spaces and parkland. Created initially as the lungs of the new industrial cities, parkland rapidly became the location for pitches for soccer, cricket and rugby, bowling greens and tennis

---

1. Holt, R., *Sport and Society in Modern France*, London, Macmillan (1981), p. 18.
2. Donnelly, P., "The Paradox of Parks, The Politics of Recreational Land Use Before and After the Mass Trespass", *Leisure Studies*, Vol. 5.2 (1986); Shoard, M., *This Land is Our Land, The Struggle for Britain's Countryside*, London, Grafton Books (1987); Holt (1981) op. cit.; and Gorn E.J. & Goldstein, W., *A Brief History of American Sports*, New York, Hill & Wang (1993).

courts.[1] In the mid-twentieth century, government intervention reflected the growing concern among physical educators and health professionals with the consequences of an increasingly sedentary lifestyle. More recently, governments have become more aware of the health issues associated with increasing drug use in sport. As will be discussed in more detail below, government concern is not limited to the use of performance enhancing drugs in competitive sport, but also encompasses the increasing prevalence of drug use in activities such as body building.

A third motive for government involvement relates to the attempt by government to use sport as a means of social integration. In Britain, sport was seen as a vehicle for instilling discipline among urban working class males, with schools being encouraged in the early part of this century to include physical training and military drill as part of the curriculum. In the 1950s and early 1960s, the traditional fear of the destabilising potential of the urban working class was reflected in a series of reports which sought to address the problem of "too much leisure". The Wolfenden Report for example, published in 1960, suggested that there was an association between the shortage of sports facilities and the rise in delinquency. More recently, the British Government responded to a series of serious urban riots in the early 1980s with the provision of more recreational facilities and the initiation by the Sports Council of the Action Sport Project which was designed to put sports leaders into local communities with the aim of fostering the integration of disaffected social groups. Public investment in sport has also been used in Northern Ireland in an attempt to bridge the sectarian divisions in the province although, in general, these policy efforts have only tended to fuel the exploitation of sport by sectarian interests. From the late 1960s the Canadian Government has also attempted to use sport to bridge the gap between its anglophone and francophone communities with, at best, mixed results.

The expectation that sport can provide a focus for community regeneration or development is widespread. In France, for example, the Vichy government of the wartime period identified sport, particularly gymnastics, as a means of "social discipline and a means of regenerating French youth".[2] An awareness of the serious risk of social problems as a result of social tensions in the suburbs of some cities led the French Government in the 1980s to seek solutions through investment in sports facilities and programmes.[3] Similar examples may be drawn from Australia and the United States where the strength of the "muscular Christian" movement in the nineteenth century established a

---

1. See Cuneen, C. "Hands Off Parks, The Provision of Parks and Playgrounds" in Roe, J. (ed.), *Twentieth Century Sydney, Studies in Urban and Social History*, Sydney, Hale & Iremonger (1980); Crantz G., *The Politics of Park Design, A History of Urban Parks in America*, Cambridge, MA, MIT Press (1982).
2. Holt (1981), op. cit., p. 58.
3. Poujol, G.,"Leisure Politics and Policies in France" in Bramham, P. et al (eds.), *Leisure Policy in Europe*, London, CAB International (1993) p. 23.

21

strong association between sport and recreation on the one hand and the maintenance of social integration and stability on the other.[1]

Governments have also intervened in sport when there was a need to strengthen the military preparedness of the country. In the late 1930s and early 1940s many governments introduced legislation or programmes in an attempt to improve the level of fitness among potential conscripts. This fourth policy motive is evident not just among the major European governments but also in Australia and Canada. For all these governments their interest in sport was secondary to their pre-occupation with reducing the high rejection rates of military recruits that they experienced during the first world war.[2]

A fifth motive for government involvement in sport is the use of international sporting success as a convenient and relatively cheap way of enhancing the country's prestige and as a means of expanding the repertoire of diplomatic tools available to government. It is in relation to these two overlapping motives that the temptation is strongest among governments, at worst, to sanction the use of drugs or, at best, to turn a blind eye to their use. Governments are increasingly aware of the high media profile of international sport and the potential of sport to reflect and enhance, but also to undermine, the prestige of the country. For many western European and North American countries the startling success of the then German Democratic Republic (GDR) and Soviet Union in the early 1960s was a significant challenge to the comfortable assumptions of western sporting superiority and prompted a series of debates about the threat to national prestige resulting from communist domination of major sports events. The concern with the decline in sporting performance relative to the German Democratic Republic and the Soviet Union was one of the factors that led Britain's Labour Government to appoint an Advisory Sports Council in the mid 1960s. It also prompted one of the rare interventions by the United States federal government in sport when, exasperated at the inability of the American sports bodies to organise themselves effectively for Olympic competition, it supported the passage by Congress of the Amateur Sports Act in 1978.

While the dramatic improvement in the performance of sportsmen and women from communist countries was important in providing a source of

---

1. See Boag, A., "Recreation Participation Survey, Activities Done Away from Home" in Department of Arts, Sport, the Environment, Tourism and Territories, *Ideas for Australian Recreation, Commentaries on the Recreation Participation Surveys*, Canberra, Australian Government Publishing Service (1989) and Cashman, R., *Paradise for Sport, The Rise of Organised Sport in Australia*, Melbourne, Oxford University Press (1995), p. 57, for comments on Australian policy; Lewis, G. "The Muscular Christian Movement", *Journal of Health, Physical Education and Recreation*, No. 5 (1966); Gorn & Goldstein, op. cit. (1993), Crantz, op. cit. (1982), p. 231 and Swanson, R.A. "The Acceptance and Influence of Play in American Protestantism, *Quest*, Vol.11, 1968 regarding the United States.
2. See Houlihan, B., *Sport, Policy and Politics, A Comparative Analysis*, London, Routledge (1997), Chapter 3.

motivation in many countries, for others the motivation lay more in the perceived need to enhance the profile of the country on the international stage. Especially for former colonies, the problems of establishing an identity within the international community were substantial. In Canada, for example, from the early 1960s the government, through the Fitness and Amateur Sport Act 1961, sought to achieve the dual aim of improving the level of fitness of the general population and meeting the government's "concern about national prestige and the success of elite athletes".[1] By the 1970s, the Canadian Government had established a dominant presence within the organisations responsible for elite sport development often using specialist task forces to target particular problems, events or sports. France adopted a similar interventionist policy when, in 1984, the government decided to restructure the administration of sport and give responsibility for elite development to the Ministry of Youth and Sport.

One of the clearest examples of the deliberate exploitation of sport for purposes of international prestige or diplomatic advantage concerns the former German Democratic Republic. This is also one of the clearest illustrations of government-sanctioned drug use by athletes and is a powerful reminder of the extent to which governments are tempted to treat sport and sportsmen and women as instruments for the achievement of non-sports policy objectives. The nascent GDR Government quickly recognised the utility of sport in helping to fulfil the twin policy objectives of, first, obtaining diplomatic recognition as an independent state and not simply the Soviet zone of Germany and, second, reconstructing East German culture following the nazi period.

The East German Government established a powerful sports bureaucracy under the control of the Deutscher Turn und Sports Bund (DTSB) whose long-serving president, Manfred Ewald, was also the president of the GDR's national Olympic committee. The initial emphasis of sports policy was on the contribution of sport to "the democratic revival of our nation".[2] However, during the 1950s, the emphasis began to shift from the development of mass participation in sport as a basis for civic re-education to the cultivation of elite success as a focus for the emergence of a new East German national identity. The elite sport policy was intended to realise three objectives: first, the achievement of diplomatic recognition; second, the enhancement of the status of the GDR within the communist bloc; and third, the demonstration

---

1. Franks, C.E.S. & Macintosh, D., "The Evolution of Federal Government Policies Toward Sport and Culture in Canada, A Comparison" in Theberge, N. & Donnelly, P., *Sport and the Sociological Imagination*, Fort Worth, Texas Christian University Press (1984); Macintosh, D. and Hawes, D., *Sport and Canadian Diplomacy*, Toronto, McGill-Queen's University Press (1994); Helmes, R.C., "Ideology and Social Control in Canadian Sport, A Theoretical Review", in *Sport and the Sociocultural Process*, (3rd ed.), Hart, M. & Birrell, W.C., Dubuque Iowa, Brown & Co. (1981).
2. Quoted in Hardman, K., "The Development of Physical Education in the German Democratic Republic", *Physical Education Review*, Vol. 3.2 (1980), p. 124.

to non-communist countries of the superiority of the communist system.[1] Elite sport success and membership of sports organisations such as the IOC and the major international federations were central to the GDR strategy regarding diplomatic recognition. Sustained elite success by its "diplomats in tracksuits"[2] made it increasingly difficult for the Olympic movement and the major international federations to ignore the claims of the GDR to be treated as a country distinct from the Federal Republic of Germany.

Table 1.1: East Germany's Olympic success: 1968-88

Year	Gold	Silver	Bronze	Position in medals table
1968	9	9	7	5th
1972	20	23	23	3rd
1976	40	25	25	2nd
1980	47	37	42	2nd (boycott by USA and others)
1984	Los Angeles games boycotted by GDR and others			
1988	37	35	29	2nd

From the late 1950s to the late 1980s, athletes from the GDR dominated many sports events producing, for example, seventy-seven European champions in track and field and numerous Olympic champions (see Table 1.1). Elite success was established and maintained through the employment of almost 600 full-time coaches working within an elaborate structure of specialist sports schools and colleges at a cost estimated at approximately 1.5% to 2% of Gross Domestic Product. Following reunification, the performance of former GDR athletes declined sharply. In women's swimming, which the East Germans dominated for much of the post-war period, their success dipped abruptly in the early 1990s. Whereas in the 1986 World Championships the GDR swimmers won twenty-four medals of which thirteen were gold, the performance of former East German women swimmers in the 1991 World Championships resulted in only six medals, none of which was gold. It is now widely acknowledged that systematic state-sanctioned drug abuse made a substantial contribution to the GDR's sporting (and diplomatic) success.[3] Such was the scale and the effectiveness of the doping programme that

1. Sutcliffe, P.,"The German Democratic Republic, an Overview", in Hardman, K. (ed.), *Physical Education and Sport under Communism*, Manchester, Manchester University Press (1988).
2. Comment made by GDR officials to their athletes departing for competition abroad. Quoted in Strenk, A., "Diplomats in Tracksuits, The Role of Sports in the Foreign Policy of the German Democratic Republic", *Journal of Sport and Social Issues*, spring/summer, Vol. 4.1 (1980).
3. See Berendonk, B., *Doping Dokumente, Von der Forschung zum Betrug*, Berlin, Springer-Verlag (1991). A summary of evidence is provided in English in Franke, W.W. & Berendonk, B., "Hormonal doping and androgenization of athletes, a secret program of the German Democratic Republic government", *Clinical Chemistry*, Vol. 43.7, pp. 1262-79 (1997).

one senior GDR sports official was reported as observing that "Drug-taking was the only field in which the planned economy really functioned".[1]

A similar picture of substantial state use of sport as a diplomatic resource can be found within a wide number of countries. The former Soviet Union and the United States both demonstrate a long history of government use of sport for diplomatic ends. Both countries used sport as a surrogate for their ideological rivalry, as a way of attempting to generate good relations with potential supporters and allies, and as a way of cementing links with their allies. Canada helped shape Commonwealth policy towards South Africa over apartheid and used sports development aid to poorer countries as a way of achieving its leadership on policy within the Commonwealth Heads of Government Meetings.[2] Australia too was not averse to using sport for diplomatic purposes. For example, Prime Minister Menzies encouraged the Australian Cricket Board of Control to undertake a cricket tour of the West Indies in the mid 1950s in order to enhance his standing in the Commonwealth.[3]

The final example of the range of motives that prompt government intervention in sport concerns the contribution that sport can make to economic regeneration. During the economic depression of the 1930s, the United States and Canada provided the clearest examples of the development of public works projects as a form of employment generation, many of which made valuable contributions to the sports infrastructure of communities. However, the benefits for sport and recreation were inadvertent rather than part of a planned sports resources strategy. More recently, sports investment has been seen by governments as making a valuable contribution to the local and the national economy. At the local level, stadium development has, for many years, featured as an element of a number of urban regeneration schemes.[4] In the United States urban parks and recreation facilities were advocated as a way to revitalise neighbourhoods economically and stimulate the surrounding business district.[5] It has also been noted that in Canada both the federal and provincial governments were providing major subsidies for prestigious stadium developments on the grounds that the policy "provides

---

1. Quoted in *The Times*, newspaper (UK), 16 January 1991, p. 40.
2. Macintosh, D., "Sport and the State, The Case of Canada" in Landry, F. (ed.) *Sport .... The Third Millennium*, Sainte-Foy, Les Presse de l'Université de Laval (1991); see also Macintosh, D. and Hawes, D., op. cit. (1994).
3. Cashman, R., op. cit. (1995).
4. See for example Baade, R. and Dye, R "Sports Stadiums and Area Development, A Critical Review, *Economic Development Quarterly*, 2 (August) pp. 265-75, (1988); Johnson, A.T. "The sports franchise relocation issue and public policy responses", in *Government and sport, the public policy issues*, Johnson, A.T. & Frey, J.H. (eds.) Totowa, NJ, Rowman and Allenheld (1985). Johnson, A.T, *Minor league baseball and local economic development*, Chicago, University of Illinois Press (1993); Reiss, S.A. "City Games, The Evolution of American Urban Society and the Rise of Sports", Urbana, Ill., University of Illinois Press (1989) for discussions of the phenomenon in the United States and McCormack, G., "The Price of Affluence, The Political Economy of Japanese Leisure", *New Left Review*, No. 189, pp. 121-34 (1991) for a discussion of Japan.
5. Crantz, op.cit., (1982), p. 208.

jobs and incentives for profits for the private sector as well as stimulating the local economy by bringing tourists and spectators to the community".[1]

In the United States and Canada in particular, but also in Britain, Japan, Germany and France, the longer established motive of civic "boosterism" (the development of major sports facilities as civic status symbols) has been augmented by a recognition of the potential economic return of major stadium and indoor sports facility development. At a national level the perception of hosting major sports events as a drain on public expenditure and as requiring substantial and often long-term subsidy has been replaced by a perception of events such as the World Cup and the Olympic Games as significant sources of inward investment in the form of tourism expenditure and as a net benefit to the economy. In Britain, it is estimated that the annual value of sports tourism to the economy is £1.5 billion. For the city of Sheffield the first round matches of the Euro '96 soccer competition generated around £5.8 million of expenditure. It was calculated that the 26 000 supporters who visited the city during the ten day period spent between £50 and £100 each day. It is estimated by the Australian Tourist Commission that the Sydney Olympic Games will attract an additional 2.1 million visitors between 1994 and 2000 due to the city's raised profile, and contribute over 4 billion Australian dollars to an aspect of the economy which already, in 1993, accounted for 11% of Australia's exports. This expectation is based on assessments of Australia's previous experience in bidding for and hosting major sports events. For example, it was estimated that the hosting of the 1987 America's Cup generated expenditure of 464 million Australian dollars and the equivalent of 9 500 full-time jobs. Even Brisbane's failed bid for the 1992 Olympic Games provided a significant boost to the local economy as it focused "world-wide attention on Australia, its tourism potential, its excellent sporting facilities and its professional sports administration".[2]

With the growing perception that the hosting of major events is no longer a financial burden has come the parallel perception that the chances of a successful bid are greater if a country has a strong sporting elite. The desire to host major events thus becomes one more pressure on national sports organisations and government agencies to "guarantee" elite success. One clear policy adopted by an increasing number of governments is to fund the establishment of an elite training centre. The Australian Institute of Sport at Canberra has become the model for many countries and similar centres now exist or are planned in Canada (Ottawa), the United States (Colorado Springs), the United Kingdom (Sheffield), France (Paris), the Netherlands (Arnhem) and Ireland (Limerick). Unfortunately a number of these centres, including those in Ottawa and Canberra, have been tainted with drug abuse scandals,

---

1. Macintosh, D., op. cit., (1991), p. 271.
2. Department of Sport, *Recreation and Tourism*, Annual report 1986-87, p. 49 (1987).

reflecting in large part, the intense pressure of expectations that these elite institutes are under.

Overall, the main conclusion is not just to draw attention to the increasing range of motives that have prompted greater government involvement in sport, but rather to emphasise the greater intensity of involvement. Governments in general have moved from a position where they were content to approach policy development and implementation through a process of consultation or negotiation with relatively independent national sports organisations, to a position where governments are much more directive and also more likely to introduce state agencies into the policy area. One concern must be the capacity of national sports organisations to remain effective actors in the policy process: a problem compounded by the increasing prominence of commercial interests in sport.

Sport, business and money

The intensification of government interest and involvement in sports policy is matched only by the similar surge in involvement in sport by business, a development which has brought clear rewards but also problems. It is the growth in the involvement of media businesses that best illustrates the increasing commercialisation of sport. Sport has always been an important element in the schedules of radio and television companies, but it is from the mid 1960s that the relationship began to change from one of considerable mutual benefit to one best described as mutual interdependence or symbiosis. The transformation of the relationship is partly the result of technological innovation (the development of geostationary satellites and the capacity for live broadcasts of foreign sports events), partly the effective marketing of international, and especially Olympic, sport as national or ideological clashes, and partly as a result of the success of the Olympics in attracting a huge audience, but one with the higher proportion of female, younger and more affluent viewers sought by advertisers.[1] The importance of sports to the major broadcasting companies is easily illustrated through an examination of the escalation in fees paid for the television rights to the Olympic Games. The European broadcasting companies negotiating through the European Broadcasting Union (EBU) paid US$ 670000 for the rights to the 1960 games in Rome; US$ 1.7 million for the 1972 rights; US$ 19 million in 1984; and US$ 90 million for the rights to the Barcelona games in 1992. There is currently no sign that the fee ceiling has been reached as the EBU has just agreed a figure of US$ 350 million for the Sydney 2000 games as part of a US$ 1442 billion deal securing the broadcasting rights for the five winter and summer games between 2000 and 2008. A similar escalation in the scale of

---

1. Klatell, D.A. & Marcus, N., *Sports for Sale, Television, Money and the Fans*, New York, Oxford University Press (1988); Geraghty, C., Simpson, P. & Whannel, G.,"Tunnel Vision, Television's World Cup" in Tomlinson, A. & Whannel, G. (eds.) *Off the Ball, The Football World Cup*, London, Pluto Press (1986).

fees that television companies have been willing to pay is evident in the United States where the rights to the 1960 Rome games were purchased for a mere US$ 400000. By 1972 the fees had increased to US$ 225 million, rising to US$ 401 million in 1992 and most recently to US$ 793 million for the Sydney games and US$ 2.3 billion for the 2004, 2006 and 2008 games.[1]

It is not only in the rapid increase in broadcasting fees that the greater prominence of business in sport is evident. Sponsorship contracts with individual athletes, clubs and leagues provide further evidence of the depth of the commercialisation of sport. Multi-million pound sponsorship contracts for a small number of elite sportsmen and women are no longer a rarity. Boris Becker, for example, was reputedly paid £24 million by Puma to promote their products and Tiger Woods received US$ 40 million to promote Nike. Soccer clubs are now able to negotiate lucrative sponsorship deals with major companies such as Opel who paid £ 2.2 million to advertise on the shirts of the German soccer club Bayern Munich. Sponsorship of complete leagues is also common, with the brewers Bass sponsoring the English soccer Premier League for four years at a cost of £12 million. While sponsorship is estimated to be growing at about 10% each year, the distribution of income is highly uneven in terms of the sports that benefit, the level of sport that benefits and the regions of the world that benefit. Some sports are less attractive to sponsors. Soccer, track and field, motor racing, tennis and golf are among the main beneficiaries of sponsorship and television revenue. In Britain, tobacco sponsorship of field hockey ended because the sport failed to attract a mass television audience. Squash was dropped by the tobacco company Benson and Hedges, one of the major sponsors of sport, because the image of the sport was considered inappropriate for the product. As the sales promotion manager for Benson and Hedges observed "I always felt I was in the wrong place. You could have a cigarette when playing golf or cricket and even the hockey crowd were a cosmopolitan bunch who enjoyed the odd drink and a cigarette. Squash was more obsessive."[2]

Even those sports that are regular beneficiaries of sponsorship find that business is highly selective in the aspects of the sport they support. In track and field, finding sponsorship for youth competition, regional events and even national championships is difficult. Sponsors are also generally keener on supporting sprint and middle distance track events than field events and generally prefer men's to women's events. More worrying is the fact that, with one or two minor exceptions, sponsorship flows to sports, events and athletes in the more affluent parts of the world. Athletes in poorer countries often have to rely on the meagre sports development budgets of Olympic Solidarity (currently US$ 121.9 million for the period 1997-2000) or the major federations such as the IAAF. Alternatively, poorer athletes rely on the

---

1. Neither the figures for the sale of the US rights nor those for the sale of the European rights have been moderated to take account of inflation.
2. Quoted in Wilson, N., *The Sports Business, The Men and the Money*, London, Judy Piatkus (1988). p.163.

provision of sports scholarships, often provided by universities in the United States, or, if they play soccer, transfer to European and Japanese clubs.

According to the IAAF, the gap between rich and poor countries in relation to sport has three primary dimensions: elite programmes, development planning, and programmes for mass participation. In addition there are also substantial deficiencies in the areas of sports science and medicine, qualified coaches and officials, equipment and facilities and opportunities for competition.[1] Very few countries are able to offer a substantial proportion of the full range of summer Olympic sports, with the poorer countries frequently offering only one or two to any significant level of competition. The degree of inequality of participation at the highest levels of competition is easily illustrated by reference to recent Olympic Games. At the Los Angeles games in 1984, only sixteen countries entered athletes in sixteen or more sports while ninety countries had athletes participating in five or fewer events, of which seventy-eight were developing countries. The pattern was repeated at Seoul where sixty-three national Olympic committees, overwhelmingly in developing countries, entered athletes in fewer than ten events.[2]

The striking flood of money into sport in the richer developed countries and the equally striking lack of even the most basic sports infrastructure for the majority of the world's population have consequences for doping and anti-doping policy. For the rich countries, leagues, clubs and athletes, the fear of failure and the loss of the attendant sponsorship puts enormous pressure on athletes, their coaches and managers to use whatever measures are necessary to sustain their current high level of success. Few of the major commercial sports seem prepared to address the issue or use their resources to give a lead on the issue of doping, for example through education and the provision of information. Rather than necessarily indicating a lack of interest in the issue, it might also be a reflection of the tenuous control that a number of federations, both domestic and international, exert over their commercial clubs. The reluctance of clubs to co-operate is often the result of their unwillingness to risk the loss of the services of star team members through suspension. Clubs consequently will exert pressure for financial penalties or short bans even for serious offences such as drug taking. This is most clearly the case in the United States where commercialisation is integral to most sport and where the major sports leagues, including basketball and football, have been most noticeable in their reluctance to impose substantial bans on drug abusers. However, much the same may also be said of the increasingly commercial English soccer where there is a preference for regarding positive drug tests as a signal for counselling and medical advice, albeit during a period of suspension for the player, rather than a firmer punishment which would be likely in other sports.

---

1. Wangemann, B. "Report to the IAAF development department", London, IAAF (1988).
2. Anthony, D. "The North-South and East-West Axes of Development in Sport, Can the Gaps be Bridged?" in Landry, F. et al (eds.) Sport, The Third Millennium, Sainte-Foy, Les Presse de l' Universitè de Laval (1993).

A further consequence of the wealth now available in some sports is that athletes and their coaches and managers will fight hard to avert any threat to their income from sport. One of the most significant problems facing national sports organisations and their international federations is the risk of costly legal defences of their decisions on positive doping results. Most national sports organisations (NSOs), even in affluent countries, are not rich bodies and few could withstand the imposition of modest damages should an appeal against a ban be successful and it is debatable whether many have the resources to underwrite the cost of a sustained legal challenge.

Although the situation of athletes from poorer countries may appear different, it is in many respects the same as that of their rich counterparts. However, for those on sports scholarships or with contracts with European or Japanese soccer clubs, the fear is the loss of the opportunity to break through into the elite or to retain membership once it has been achieved. As a result of these pressures, the use of drugs is not a problem confined to a particular group of athletes but is a ubiquitous problem in modern commercialised sport.

Sport, health and personal glory

The rapid growth and intensification of government and commercial interest in sport has added greatly to the pressures facing sportsmen and women in high level competition. Yet, significant though these changes undoubtedly are, there have been other developments which have been equally critical in shaping the character of modern sport. Of especial note is the growth in the cult of the body. Generally, it has been possible to equate participation in sport with good health and fitness. There have, of course, been notable qualifications to this loose equation. There has been a long-standing concern about the level of risk of injury in some, usually full contact, sports such as American football, rugby union and rugby league. There is also an emerging concern with the deliberate over-training of athletes especially in sports such as female gymnastics, where the most intensive period of training and competition takes place during puberty.

More recently the ability to generalise about the complementarity of sports participation and good health has been questioned by those social analysts who see sport as increasingly incorporated into consumer culture which encourages a high degree of self-absorption and a pre-occupation with an idealised version of femininity and masculinity. Much of the recent analysis focuses on the effects of modernity on the female body and the way in which self-perception of women is influenced by a culture and by a sports and leisure industry that values women's bodies in terms of male desire.[1] The current western cultural stigmatisation of fatness is frequently seen as being the

---

1. Boskind-Lodhal, M. "Cinderella Stepsisters, A Feminist Perspective on Anorexia Nervosa" in *Signs*, Vol. 2.2, pp. 342-56; MacLeod, S. *The Art of Starvation*, London, Verso (1981).

root cause of eating disorders such as anorexia nervosa and responsible for the growth in obsessive concerns with fitness. "Western culture associates fat bodies with indiscipline and indulgence; by contrast, thin bodies symbolise asceticism and self-control."[1] Being thin and fit is one way of publicly demonstrating one's right to a place in modern society, with the wearing of sports clothing in non-sporting situations being a further way of demonstrating one's credentials for membership in today's world. Although the feminist analysis has its critics, there is a more general acceptance that within contemporary culture the image of women's bodies constructed by men, a climate of narcissism and a more general idealisation of the female body has helped to foster an increase in participation in fitness activities. This is motivated less by a desire for empowerment and the building of self-esteem or a desire to be fit to play sport and more by an inability to cope with the pressures of contemporary culture.[2]

The incidence of sports participation as pathological behaviour is not limited to women. Although less well researched, it is clear that men are not immune to the pressures of modern society. For men the development of an idealised physique is an expression of empowerment and self-confidence within a society that, on the one hand, has given economic and political priority to the individual over society, but, on the other hand appears increasingly dismissive of individual worth. For an increasing, yet still small, number of young men the path to their desired physique involves not only hours on the fitness equipment of the gymnasium but also the use of anabolic steroids. Although the volume of empirical data is small, the data that exist indicate that a surprisingly high proportion of steroid users have a cosmetic and non-sport motive. A 1988 study showed that 2% out of a total sample of 1 010 college students admitted taking steroids.[3] More interestingly, just under half (42%) of the steroid users claimed they were taking the drug for the sake of appearance or body building. In Britain it is reported that there is "anecdotal evidence to suggest that anabolic steroid abuse is higher in areas with a macho culture, ample male leisure time (that is unemployment), low self-esteem and proximity to (...) a suitable location to parade the results of your body building".[4]

The emergence of steroid abusers who take the drugs for reasons of vanity and self-esteem rather than to gain a competitive edge may be deemed a further consequence of the spread of drug abuse in sport. However, it also needs to be seen in the context of an increasingly pill-dependent society. It is

---

1. Rojek, C., *Decentring Leisure, Rethinking Leisure Theory*, London, Sage (1995), p. 63.
2. Bruch, H. *The Golden Cage, The Enigma Anorexia Nervosa*, Cambridge, Mass., Harvard University Press (1977).
3. Pope, H.G., Katz, D.L. & Champoux, R. "Affective and psychotic symptoms associated with anabolic steroid use", *American Journal of Psychiatry*, Vol. 51, pp. 487-90 (1988).
4. George, A. "The Anabolic Steroids and Peptide Hormones", in *Drugs in Sport* (2nd. ed.), Mottram, D.R. (ed.) (1996).

unrealistic to expect athletes to insulate themselves from a culture which expects pharmacists and doctors to be able to supply medicines for all their ills whether physical or psychological. It is also unrealistic to ignore the importance of legitimate drugs in the intensely scientific training regimes of most, if not all, elite athletes in the 1990s. The use of dietary supplements and vitamins is routine, and the willingness of athletes and their coaches to experiment with untested herbal concoctions defies common sense but also indicates the desire, indeed desperation, of many athletes to find a means of giving them an edge over their rivals. "By the time [athletes] have made the pros, most athletes have been given so many pills, salves, injections, potions, by amateur and pro coaches, doctors and trainers, to pick them up, cool them down, kill pain, enhance performance, reduce anxiety, that there isn't much they won't sniff, spread, stick in or swallow to get bigger or smaller, or to feel good (sic)".[1]

Conclusion

The feeling of shock that most sports enthusiasts experience when another drug scandal is revealed is not simply the reaction to another example of duplicitous behaviour. It is also a feeling of being personally cheated; the private emotions that a spectacular medal-winning performance generated have been publicly betrayed. It is possible to mock the disillusioned spectator or participant as being naive in expecting all sportsmen and women to adhere to a higher moral code than the rest of society. However, such a response would be churlish as it would fail to acknowledge the salience of sport in modern society and to belittle the motives of the majority who devote their time to sport, much of it given without financial reward, as coaches, administrators and participants to promote sport as an oasis within society where one can aspire to a higher morality. Yet, while such aspirations are laudable they must be tempered by an awareness of the changes that have taken place in the context of sport over the last thirty years. While it is still possible to expect sportsmen and women to subscribe to high moral standards, it is unreasonable to expect them to be immune from social change. The challenge facing sports organisations and governments in attempting to eradicate drug abuse is an increasingly daunting one. Governments are often ambiguous on the question of drug abuse and commercial interests frequently appear content to ignore the issue. Against this background, sports drug agencies have to cope with increasingly sophisticated drugs, the rapid growth in elite competition and a high level of geographical mobility of sportsmen and women.

---

1. Lipsyte, R. "Baseball and Drugs", *The Nation*, May 25th (1985), p. 613.

Chapter 2

The evolution of doping

Early examples of drug use

It is a commonplace to state that doping, along with other forms of cheating, is not new. Yet it seems necessary to preface any discussion with this reminder as there is a tendency for many involved in sport as spectators, participants, coaches or officials to imagine a past sporting world dominated by the noble of spirit and the pure of heart. The long history of doping should put modern policymakers on their guard against seeking an easy solution to the problem. But the history of doping does not just demonstrate the continuity or intractability of the problem in sport, it clarifies the modern dimensions of the problem which require ingenuity and commitment from policy makers.

In general, wherever and whenever the outcome of a sporting competition has involved status, money or other property, attempts have been made to seek an advantage through doping. From the standpoint of the end of the twentieth century, the methods and substances seem crude and of questionable value, but the motive provides an indelible link between the centuries. In the third century BC, Greek athletes were taking varieties of mushroom to improve their performance.[1] Greek athletes were also reported as training on special diets which included dried figs; Egyptians had confidence in the properties of the ground rear hooves of the Abyssinian ass while Roman gladiators were reported to take stimulants to overcome fatigue.[2]

More recently, during the nineteenth century there were many accounts of athletes using a variety of substances to enhance their performance, including strychnine, nitro-glycerine, opium, alcohol and caffeine.[3] In the mid-nineteenth century there were reports of competitive swimmers in Amsterdam taking an opium-based drug. In 1869 there were reports of cycling coaches preparing heroin and cocaine mixtures for their riders in order to increase their endurance during continuous 144-hour races. Belgian cyclists were alleged to have been taking ether-soaked tablets, the French took caffeine tablets while the British were allegedly relying on a range of drugs including

---

1. Puffer, J., "The Use of Drugs in Swimming" in *Clinical Sports Medicine*, Vol. 5.77 (1986).
2. Finley, D.F. & Plecket, H. W. op. cit.; Hanley, D.F. "Drug and Sex Testing, Regulations for International Competition", *Clinical Sports Medicine*, Vol. 2, pp. 13-17 (1983); Meer, J. "Drugs and Sports" in Snyder, S.H. (ed.), *The Encyclopedia of Psychoactive Drugs*, New York, Chelsea House, (1987).
3. Puffer, op. cit.

strychnine, heroin, brandy and cocaine as well as inhaling pure oxygen.[1] It was inevitable that the administration of these and other equally dangerous drugs would lead to a fatality. The death of the cyclist Arthur Linton in 1886 may be the first recorded death of an athlete from an overdose of drugs. However, the last twenty years of the nineteenth century was a period during which some very dangerous drugs such as strychnine were tested to the limits of human tolerance.[2] Despite the publicity it generated, the death did little if anything to dissuade drug users. Reports of doping continued to appear throughout the remaining years of the century.

Drug use in the twentieth century

Apart from the American athlete, Tom Hicks, and his infamous involvement in the marathon at the 1904 St. Louis Olympics where he collapsed following the use of a strychnine-brandy cocktail, the early part of the twentieth century was not marked by any major escalation or development in drug use. There continued to be examples of the use of crude drugs and preparations, often administered more in hope rather than with any certainty that they would aid performance. In the 1930s, for example, there were reports of athletes using a mixture of powdered gelatine and orange juice in the expectation of enhanced performance.[3] The next phase in the history of drug use came later in the century when the synthesis and mass production of drugs became more common (see Table 2.1). However, the crucial catalyst for the widespread use of drugs in sport came with the extensive and frequently unregulated experimentation with drugs during the second world war. The use of amphetamines and steroids in particular by the military not only greatly increased scientific knowledge about the properties of the various drugs but also demonstrated the widespread opportunities for the use of the drugs outside a therapeutic context.

Amphetamines

In the early post-war period evidence about drug abuse continued to accumulate, as indeed did the deaths. Amphetamine and its derivatives rapidly replaced the earlier cruder preparations, such as strychnine, as the preferred drug of athletes, especially those involved in explosive and endurance events. Not surprisingly, throughout the 1950s cyclists continued to be identified as the main group of athletes thought to be heavily involved in drug abuse, though drug taking was also considered to be rife in professional

---

1. Voy, R., *Drugs, Sport and Politics, The Inside Story about Drug Use in Sport and its Political Cover-up*, Champaign, Ill., Leisure Press (1991).
2. Dyment, P.G., "Drug Use and the Adolescent Athlete", Pediatric Annals, Vol. 13, p. 602, (1984). Donohoe, T. and Johnson, N., *Foul Play, Drug Abuse in Sports*, Oxford, Blackwell (1986), suggest that Linton did not die during or close to competition but in fact died many years later from typhoid.
3. Asken, M.J. *Dying to Win, The Athlete's Guide to Safe and Unsafe Drugs in Sport*, Washington DC, Acropolis Books (1988).

Table 2.1: History of drug use and doping practices in sport (major drugs and practices only)

Drug	Approximate date of discovery	First use in sport	Extent of use	Major sports affected	Peak of use	Current level of use
Amphetamines	1920s	1940s	Heavy use between the mid 1950s and the late 1970s	Cycling, American football	Late 1960s to early 1980s	Light, due to ease of identification and availability of alternatives
Ephedrine and related stimulants	c1940s	1970s	Heavy use from mid 1970s to the present	Most Olympic sports and many major team sports	Yet to be reached	Heavy
Caffeine	Pre-19th century	Early 19th century	Heavy in 19th century then declined, only to increase in use from 1970s to the present day in combination with ephedrine and as a diuretic	Most Olympic sports and many major team sports	19th century, then from the mid 20th century to the present	Heavy, but mainly in conjunction with other drugs
Blood doping and rEPO	Blood doping 1970s / rEPO Mid 1980s	1970s / Late 1980s	Moderate / Light in later 1980s but rising (rEPO)	Endurance sport such as long distance cycling, running, swimming and cross-country skiing	1980s / Still rising (rEPO)	Moderate / Moderate but rising (rEPO)
Barbiturates	Early 20th century	1970s	Moderate	Modern Pentathlon (shooting)	1970s	Light
Beta-blockers	1960s	1970s	Moderate use in small number of sports	Shooting, archery and snooker	Late 1980s	Moderate, but use not completely banned by IFs and IOC
Anabolic steroids and anabolic agents	1930s	1950s	Heavy between the late 1960s and the late 1980s	Most Olympic sports and many major team sports	Mid 1980s	Heavy
Cocaine	Pre-17th century	Late 19th century	Heavy between the late 1960s and the present day	American football	1980s	Moderate
Human growth hormone	Mid 1980s	Late 1980s	Moderate and mainly confined to the United States of America (?)	Body building and a similar range of sports that attract anabolic steroid users	Yet to be reached	Small but rising
Diuretics	Synthetic diuretics 1960s	1970s?	Moderate to heavy in early 1970s	Weight related sports, but all sports when used as a drug to flush others out of the body	mid 1970s	Light, due to ease of identification.

boxing and several speed-skaters became ill through the over-use of amphetamines during the 1952 Helsinki Olympics. But it was not until a series of deaths in the 1960s that sports organisations were prompted to move from a stance of condemnation and dismay to a more interventionist position. In 1960 the Danish cyclist, Knut Jensen, collapsed and died at the Rome Olympic Games during the 175-kilometres team time-trials following his use of amphetamines and nicotine acid. Jensen's two teammates, who had taken the same mixture, also collapsed but later recovered in hospital. Tom Simpson's death in the 1967 Tour de France brought on by excessive use of methamphetamine was caught on television and dramatically raised the profile of the issue in Britain. Simpson's death was followed the next year by the death of the French cyclist Yves Mottin a few days after he had won a gruelling cross-country cycling event.[1] Despite the focus of attention on the implications of the growing use of amphetamines and the increasing number of fatalities, there was also a continuing use of heroin and a steady increase in the number of deaths. The hurdler, Dick Howard, died at the Rome Olympics from heroin, the same drug that was found in the body of the boxer, Billy Bello, who died three years later.

By the mid 1930s, scientific experimentation with amphetamines had resulted in its adoption for therapeutic use, for example in the treatment of narcolepsy, but had also alerted the German military authorities to the potential uses of the drug in overcoming fatigue during combat. Evidence of the use of amphetamines in sport began to emerge in the late 1950s, with the drug beginning to become fashionable among young people as a social drug in the mid 1960s. As with all attempts to plot accurately the development and extent of drug use the history of the spread of amphetamine use in sport must be tentative. A 1984 study in the United States found that 8% of university students admitted using amphetamines within the previous twelve months with one-third of the total using the drug to enhance their sports performance.[2] Use was especially high among football players who, in the 1970s, replaced cyclists as the groups of athletes giving greatest cause for concern. Approximately two-thirds of the sample of professional football players interviewed had used amphetamines, half of whom admitted to regular use. Dosages ranged from 5 milligrams to 200 milligrams per game: dosages at the mid to upper end of this range have been associated with manic behaviour.[3] A 1984 study claimed that "amphetamines are probably

---

1. It is interesting that the long association between drug use in general and amphetamine use in particular in cycling has not led to a significant discussion about the nature of some events in the sport, such as the Tour de France and Tour d'Italia. It can be argued that the unrelenting intensity of endurance cycling makes it difficult for athletes to participate without assistance from drugs. In other words, it is the sport which is unnatural rather than the drug-using competitors.
2. Anderson, W.A. & McKeag, D.B., "The Substance Use and Abuse Habits of College Student Athletes", Research Paper No.2, General Findings, Michigan, Michigan State University (1985).
3. Mandell, A.J., Stewart, K.D. & Russo, P.V., "The Sunday Syndrome, From Kinetics to Altered Consciousness", Federal Proceedings, Vol. 40, (1981).

the principal drug misuse problem in athletics", but the early 1980s probably marked the high point of abuse as the drug began to be replaced by caffeine and steroids and also as it became much more easily detectable.[1]

Although drug use has been accused of altering the character of some sports it is probably more accurate to argue that drug use has exaggerated certain aspects of particular sports, often those aspects that already give rule makers greatest cause for concern. American football is a good example as it is a sport that many claim has been seriously undermined by the extensive abuse of drugs, such as amphetamines and steroids. At its best American football as a contact sport relies on a combination of athleticism, determination and bravery for its excitement. Yet many clubs and sportsmen involved in the sport have trodden a fine line between athleticism and aggression, determination and brutality, and between bravery and recklessness. In the early years of the sport one of the most pressing problems facing the nascent governing body for the sport was the need to control the level of violence. The high number of deaths in the 1905 season prompted President Theodore Roosevelt to call a meeting in an attempt to persuade the three major universities, Harvard, Yale and Princeton, to reform the sport. The impact of the presidential intervention was negligible as football remained an, at times, harsh and brutal sport, fulfilling the role in American society of "defining and testing physical and psychological masculinity [...] Though football carried fewer risks than military combat, players invested it with many of the same feelings".[2]

Almost one hundred years later little has changed in the social significance of the sport or in the spirit in which it is played. The effect that access to drugs has had is to make it more difficult for the sport's governing authority to ensure that the attributes of athleticism, determination and bravery are protected from those who aspire only to aggression, brutality, and recklessness. An account of the huge quantities of amphetamines taken by players on a regular basis is graphic: "Imagine what it is like to gulp down thirty pills at one time. The result is a prepsychotic paranoid rage state. A five-hour temper tantrum that produces the late hits..., the unconscionable assaults on quarterbacks that are ruining pro-football".[3] The use of steroids has much the same effect, inducing in the user what has been termed "roid rage" which is essentially an inability to control aggression. With extensive and sustained steroid use the loss of judgement is compounded by the added danger arising from the increase in bulk of the user and the consequent capacity to inflict more serious injury on opponents. Thus, rather than changing sport, drug abuse has the effect of exaggerating those elements that have long

1. Dyment, P.G., "Drugs and the Adolescent Athlete", *Pediatric Annals*, Vol. 13.8, pp. 602-604 (1984).
2. Gorn, E.J. & Goldstein, W. (1993), p. 163, op. cit.
3. Quoted in Goldman, B., op. cit. (1992), p. 52, *Federal Proceedings*, Vol. 40, (1981).

proved a threat to the integrity of the sport and the delicate balance of attributes that mark out the great spectator and participant sports.

Ephedrine and related stimulants

Ephedrine, along with pseudoephedrine and phenylpropanolamine, are examples of a family of drugs which mimic the effects of amphetamines. These "look-alike" drugs (prototypic sympathomimetic amines) are similar to amphetamines in that they are stimulants which act on the central nervous system. Drugs from within this family are present in many proprietary medicines, most commonly in cold remedies and nasal decongestants, and can be bought over the counter without a medical prescription in many countries and are usually available in combination with caffeine. They first emerged as drugs used by athletes in the 1970s when countries were achieving greater success in restricting the availability of amphetamines.

The first occasion on which the drug came to public attention was during the 1972 Munich Olympic Games when the American swimmer, Rick DeMont, tested positive for ephedrine. Despite having informed officials that he was using an anti-asthma drug (Marex) he was stripped of his gold medal for the 400-metres freestyle and was disqualified from participating in the remaining events for which he was entered. Some twelve years later the British-Canadian athlete, Ronald Angus, was given a life ban by the British Judo Federation after traces of sympathomimetic amines were found in his urine sample. The traces were from the drug whose proprietary name was Sudafed, a nasal decongestant, prescribed by his doctor. Unlike DeMont, Angus successfully appealed against the imposition of a life ban and was reinstated in time to compete in the trials for the 1984 Los Angeles Olympics.[1]

Stimulants from the sympathomimetic amine family, especially pseudoephedrine, are still regularly found in the samples of drug abusers in sport. The main problem facing the enforcers of the doping regulations is how to respond to the frequently voiced defence that the drugs were taken inadvertently as part of a cold or cough remedy bought at the local pharmacy. The challenge facing the testing authorities has been to establish a level of mild sympathomimetic amine which would distinguish between normal therapeutic use and doping. It is expected that the IOC will introduce such a reporting level in 1998. At the 1988 Olympics a British athlete was prevented from competing in a relay event due to a positive test which showed traces of pseudoephedrine in the urine sample. The athlete had previously tested negative on seven occasions but was taking ginseng. Forgo, in an experiment with ginseng capsules administered to a control group for fourteen days, found no traces of banned substances in their urine but Watt et al have drawn attention to the dangers of contaminated ginseng in many

---

1. Donohoe, T. & Johnson, N. (1986), op. cit.

commercial preparations. Linford Christie, in one memorable illustration of the problem, tested positive for an extremely small trace of pseudoephedrine at the Seoul Olympics. Christie successfully argued that the trace was due to an ingestion of a cold cure preparation where pseudoephedrine was not mentioned in the ingredients. That Christie was not banned illustrates not only the care that athletes need to exercise in taking any substance or preparation where the ingredients are not clearly listed, but also the fact that many test results for drug abuse do not produce unequivocal evidence of a doping infraction. Rather than the answer to the question "Have the federation's doping regulations been broken?" being "Yes" or "No" it is often "Maybe" or "We are not sure".

Ephedrine appears to be widely used, with cyclists being among those athletes who regularly test positive for the drug. Research undertaken in Belgium illustrates not only the pervasiveness of ephedrine abuse within cycling but also the game of "cat and mouse" that is played out between drug abusers and those attempting to eradicate doping. The test results for 4 374 cyclists were analysed between 1987 and 1994.[1] Table 2.2 shows the pattern of drug abuse over the period and the consistency with which ephedrine and norephedrine in particular occur throughout the period.

Table 2.2: Incidence of selected doping substances in cyclists 1987-94

	1987	1988	1989	1990	1991	1992	1993	1994	Total
Ephedrine	6	18	21	20	22	13	15	10	125
Norephedrine	5	26	8	14	20	7	10	7	97
Nandrolone	15	29	8	13	12	4	6	6	93
Amphetamine	8	18	13	10	11	11	9	8	88
Prolintane	2	5	1	1	3	3	6	2	23
Pseudoephedrine	0	1	2	2	3	1	6	2	17
Testosterone	1	1	2	0	0	3	4	3	14
Pemoline	0	4	2	2	0	2	3	0	13
Number of tests	230	464	550	650	587	500	637	656	4374
Number of positives*	30	70	54	50	57	39	61	40	401
% positives	13.0	15.1	9.8	7.7	9.7	7.8	9.6	6.1	9.2

* Includes refusals and fraudulent tests.
Source: adapted from Delbeke (1996)

---

1. Delbeke, F.T. "Doping in Cyclism, Results of Unannounced Controls in Flanders", *International Journal of Sports Medicine*, Vol. 17, pp. 434-438 (1996).

For the period as a whole the average figure for positives was 7.8%, which is a very high proportion and one which climbs higher when the number of refusals is added, giving an average for the period of 9.2%. More significantly, there is relatively little variation in the proportion of positive results throughout the period. The table also shows the continuing popularity of amphetamines despite the relative ease with which they can be detected. A final feature of the pattern of doping among Flemish cyclists is the incidence of multiple drug use. Particularly popular were combinations of amphetamines and ephedrine and also amphetamines in combination with steroids.

Caffeine

Caffeine has a long history of both social and medical use. Soon after the drug first appeared in central Europe in the seventeenth century, claims were quickly made regarding its success in curing a broad range of ailments including venereal disease, colds and gout. Although caffeine is present in a number of drinks the most common source is coffee and "caffeine remains the most widely consumed drug in Europe and America".[1]

The claims for caffeine's healing properties were not lost on athletes who certainly by the middle of the nineteenth century were taking substantial quantities of caffeine in the belief that it would help their sporting performance. The popularity of caffeine as an ergogenic aid was due in large part to its ease of purchase, its cheapness and its high level of public acceptability. Until comparatively recently the primary perceived utility of caffeine was as a stimulant. But, as synthetic stimulants have been developed, such as amphetamine and the sympathomimetic amines, the use of caffeine has declined. However, it also has some utility as a diuretic, a drug which can be used to flush other drugs out of the system. Even this use of caffeine is declining as more effective synthetic diuretics have been developed. Nonetheless, caffeine is still on the list produced by the IOC, but as a restricted drug rather than a banned substance, partly because of its diuretic properties but also because of the ubiquity of the drug and the plausibility of the argument that its presence in a urine sample is the result of social use rather than an attempt to cheat. The weakness of any proven significant utility of caffeine has not stopped large numbers of athletes believing that its use will improve their performance. During the 1972 marathon at the Munich Olympics, the gold medal winner, Frank Shorter, is alleged to have been given regular drinks of decarbonated Coca-Cola.[2] At the 1976 Olympic Games significant amounts of caffeine were found in the urine samples of athletes.[3] In 1984, for example, the American Federation of Cycling revealed that its team had taken

---

1. Wadler & Hainline (1989), p. 107, op. cit.
2. Brown, W.M., "Paternalism, Drugs, and the Nature of Sports", *Journal of the Philosophy of Sport*, Vol. XI, pp. 14-22 (1984).
3. Laurin, C.A. & Letorneau, G., "Medical Report on the Montreal Olympic Games", *American Journal of Sports Medicine*, Vol. 6, pp. 54-61 (1978).

caffeine suppositories before competing in the Los Angeles Olympics, while a survey undertaken by the Canadian Centre for Drug-free Sport found that 26% of a sample of 16000 11- to 18-year-olds had used caffeine to enhance performance.[1] However, as will be made clear below, for testing authorities to be concerned at the presence of caffeine in a sample, the concentration would have to be far in excess of normal social use (that is over 12 micrograms per millilitre). There have only been two athletes who have recently tested positive for concentrations of caffeine above that permitted by the IOC, an American cyclist and an Australian member of the modern pentathlon team, who both tested positive at the Seoul Olympics.[2]

Blood doping: transfusions and rEPO

Blood doping by transfusion refers to the practice of giving athletes transfusions of blood which may be their own or that of a donor. The purpose is to increase the capacity of the blood to transport oxygen to the muscles and it is based on the principle that the amount of oxygen available to the muscles is determined by the quantity of red blood cells in the body. Therefore, if the number of red blood cells can be increased, so too can the volume of oxygen transported to the muscles during competition. One form of blood doping by transfusion is to remove a volume of blood from the athlete, separate the red blood cells from the plasma and feeze-preserve the red blood cells. Following the removal of the blood the number of red blood cells in the athlete's body will gradually return to a normal level at which time the preserved red blood cells can be injected into the athlete's blood stream in time for competition.

Blood doping is especially effective in the sports that require stamina, such as long distance cycling and running, and cross-country skiing. The first rumours of this practice emerged in the early to mid 1970s and were rife during the 1976 Montreal Olympic Games where the Finnish and East German teams were the target of considerable suspicion.[3] The celebrated Finnish runner Lasse Viren, who was a specialist at the 5000 metres and 10000 metres events and won gold medals at both the 1972 and 1976 games, was questioned repeatedly about his possible involvement in blood doping by transfusion, allegations which he strenuously denied. Confirmation of the use of blood doping by transfusion came in 1981 when the Finnish steeplechaser who competed in the 1971 European Games and the Munich Olympics the following year admitted that he had undergone transfusions prior to Olympic competition. Further revelations came in the mid 1980s when eight members

---

1. Stamford, B. "Caffeine and Athletes", *Physician and Sports Medicine*, Vol. 17, pp. 193-94 (1989); Rogers, C.C. "Cyclists try caffeine suppositories", *Physician and Sports Medicine*, Vol. 13, pp. 38-40, (1985); CCDS survey reported in Graham, T.E, Rush, J.W.E. & van Soeren, M.H. "Caffeine and exercise metabolism and performance", *Canadian Journal of Applied Physiology*, Vol. 19, pp. 111-38, (1994).
2. Nehlig, A. & Derby, G. "Caffeine and Sports Activity, A Review", *International Journal of Sports Medicine*, Vol. 15, pp. 215-223 (1994).
3. Australia (1989), op. cit.

of the United States cycling team, including the winner of a gold medal and a world record holder, admitted blood doping by transfusion two days before competition in the Los Angeles Olympics where the team collected nine medals.[1] It was reported that there had been a period of silence following the games until Mark Whitehead and a colleague from the American team revealed that half of the team had received an infusion of their own or a relative's blood".[2] That the doping had been carried out under the supervision of both the team doctor and trainer made the revelations all the more shocking.

Estimating accurately the extent of blood doping is much more difficult than estimating the frequency of other forms of doping and indeed relies on admissions of use as there is currently no reliable test for the practice. It is therefore not surprising that there have been few public cases and since the mid 1980s there have been no admissions similar to those of the American cycle team. This might mean that the practice is continuing but that users are now more discreet or it might mean that the value of the practice is being questioned, at least by comparison with other forms of doping currently available.

In the last ten years the development of rEPO (recombinant erythropoietin) has provided potential blood dopers with an alternative in drug form. Erythropoietin, a synthetic drug, and human rEPO function by stimulating the production of red blood cells within the bone marrow. The identification of the properties and potential medical applications of rEPO in 1987 was followed rapidly by the first references to the use of the drug in sport. However, because of the difficulty in developing a reliable test for the drug the evidence is circumstantial rather than direct. Accusations of abuse of rEPO have again focused on cycling with a French magazine drawing attention to the large number of cyclists who had died of heart failure, one of the most common risks associated with rEPO use. One claim is that eighteen cyclists are thought to have died as a result of rEPO up to 1991 with a second claim that twelve Dutch cyclists died from cardiac failure between 1987 and 1991.[3] The advent of rEPO is causing considerable problems for anti-doping authorities and it is currently impossible to estimate with any confidence the extent of use.

Barbiturates and benzodiazepines

Barbiturates are used to suppress the central nervous system and have been in medical use for almost one hundred years. Chloral hydrate was available in

---

1. Goldman, B. (1992), op. cit.; Mottram, D.R. "Drugs in Sport" (2nd. edn.) pp. 24-5, London, E & FN Spon (1996).
2. Donohoe, T. & Johnson, N. (1986), p. 118, op. cit.
3. Robert Hartmann, writing in the *Tagesanzeiger* newspaper (Zurich) and the *Observer* newspaper, quoted in Mottram, D.R. (1996), p. 232, op. cit.

1869 and the first barbiturate derived from barbituric acid was used in clinical medicine in 1903.[1] Although barbiturates were prescribed in huge quantities in the early part of the century there was a serious concern about the capacity of the drug to create a physical and psychological dependence among users. Within medicine and within sport alternatives were sought from amongst the compounds from the benzodiazepine family which were considered as a non-addictive alternative and a set of drugs not proscribed by the IOC, although they are banned by the UIPMB, the international federation controlling the modern pentathlon and diathlon.[2] Unfortunately, the benzodiazepines have also proved to create dependence.

Within sport, barbiturates and benzodiazepines are considered to reduce anxiety, but without any loss of judgement and co-ordination, and have tended to be used most frequently to control muscle tremor in throwing sports. They could also be used in any sport where a steady hand is required, such as shooting and snooker. The most serious abuse of minor tranquillisers occurred at the Munich Olympics of 1972 where more than a quarter of competitors in the modern pentathlon had taken tranquillisers. Accurate information about trends in the use of the minor tranquillisers is unavailable but it is likely that use is declining, partly because they have been superseded by beta-blockers, discussed below, which have proved particularly popular among marksmen.

Beta-blockers

Beta-blockers are used to treat a range of medical conditions including migraine, hypertension, angina and a number of anxiety disorders. The effect of the drugs on heart rate and blood pressure make beta-blockers of little value in most sports. However, the capacity of the drugs to lower anxiety levels, steady the breathing and reduce hand and arm tremor levels have made them popular in a limited number of sports, primarily those that require a steady hand and great precision such as snooker, darts, bowls, archery and shooting. There is evidence of limited use of the drug in fencing (a combat sport) and show jumping (a high risk sport), both sports where relaxation, precision control and concentration are of value.[3]

It was during the 1980s, and largely within the Olympic sport of the modern pentathlon, that the debate about the possible misuse of the drugs was at its most intense. Modern pentathlon involves competition in a series of different sports including cross country running and shooting and because it was normal to hold these events on different days it was possible for athletes who wished to cheat to tailor their drug use to the needs of the particular sport of the day. At the 1984 Los Angeles Olympics, beta-blockers were not

1. Wadler, G.I. & Hainline, B. (1989), p.114, op. cit.
2. UIPMB (Union Internationale de Pentathlon Moderne et Biathlon).
3. Australia, op. cit., p. 25-26 (1989).

prohibited although team doctors had to notify the IOC whenever one of their team members was taking the drug. The fact that a number of team doctors were submitting notification not simply for the isolated squad member but for whole teams involved in shooting events and in the modern pentathlon sounded the alarm bells in the IOC Medical Commission.[1] The use of beta-blockers was confirmed also through the IOC's own testing procedures which identified a number of positives among athletes involved in the modern pentathlon. Because the drug was not on the IOC list of banned substances the names of the athletes testing positive were not revealed. However, the incident not only concerned the IOC but prompted the UIPMB to lobby hard for the inclusion of the beta-blockers on the IOC list. In addition, the Secretary General of UIPMB insisted on the release of the names of the countries whose doctors had notified the IOC of the use of beta-blockers by their teams. Eventually, in November 1984, it was announced that at least one competitor from Switzerland and one from the United States had legally used beta-blockers at the Olympic Games.[2] Attempts to thwart drug users by holding the shooting event on the same day as the cross country running only prompted athletes to select a short-acting beta-blocker.

It is not just the modern pentathlon that has been affected by controversy over the use of beta-blockers: the use of the drug in the non-Olympic sport of snooker also prompted considerable debate. Following the newspaper revelation in 1987 that the chairman of the sport's governing body, Rex Williams, had been taking beta-blockers for fifteen years, it was also revealed that a large number of elite players, including two former world champions, had used or were currently using beta-blockers. The governing body of the sport, the World Professional Billiards and Snooker Association, eventually agreed to ban the drug but continue to allow its use for therapeutic purposes if there was independent medical support.

Anabolic steroids

One of the most interesting aspects of the history of drug abuse in sport is the way in which drugs, developed for scientific experimental or medical purposes, become recognised as having a value in sport and how they are gradually adapted for use within a sports context. The synthesis of anabolic steroids is especially instructive. As early as the eighteenth century scientists suspected that the testes were central to the development of male characteristics. In 1849 Berthold conducted experiments on castrated cockerels by transplanting testes to their abdominal cavity which retarded the development of the characteristics normally expected following castration. Later in the nineteenth century scientists experimented with ways of extracting the

---

1. At the 1984 Olympic Games, the entire Italian shooting team announced that they needed beta-blockers in order to take part in their events.
2. Donohoe, T. & Johnson, N. (1986), pp. 85-87, op. cit.

chemicals essential to the development of male characteristics from the testes. However, it was not until 1935 that Laqueur successfully isolated testosterone in a crystalline form.[1] Over subsequent years it became clear that testosterone was one of a family of compounds which possessed a male hormone-like activity; the name of this family of compounds is androgens. The first medical use of the new drug was in the 1930s when it was used to help the recovery of starvation victims. It was also used in the same decade for the non-medical purpose of increasing the aggressiveness and strength of German soldiers. It was not until the early 1950s that the first reports began to surface that anabolic steroids were being used by athletes. The first reports came from the Soviet Union and coincided with the country's return to Olympic competition when its spectacular success at the 1952 Helsinki games began three decades of superpower rivalry for Olympic domination of the medal table.

As the rumours of steroid use among Soviet athletes multiplied during the late 1950s, two factors coincided to accelerate the spread of steroid use in western Europe and especially in the United States. The first was the distortion of values generated by the cold war and the McCarthyite hysteria that swept America. The second factor was the willingness of a number of doctors to abuse their privileged position in society and to supply drugs to athletes. As Goldman notes, "When steroids first came on the scene there were many physicians, including the father of anabolic steroids, Dr John Ziegler, who cautiously embraced them, and willingly prescribed them to athletes for whom they were responsible...[P]atriotism was a factor as well. The feeling of these doctors was that if they could in any way help an American athlete bring home the gold, they had somehow struck a blow for freedom".[2] Ziegler became aware of the use of steroids by the Soviet team at the 1956 World Games in Moscow, where the extent of use was so great that male athletes had to be catheterised in order to pass urine as the use of steroids had enlarged their prostate gland making the passing of urine in the normal way difficult or impossible.[3] As a result, and in "conjunction with the Ciba Pharmaceutical Company, Zeigler (sic) developed anabolic steroids for use by weightlifters".[4] The new drug, Dianabol, was an attempt to develop a steroid which had reduced side effects associated with the use of straight testosterone. Dianabol rapidly became established in American, and later European, gymnasiums as the preferred drug among athletes. As the number of early anabolic steroid users began to win events, the word soon spread that the route to competitive success was through the use of the new drug.

1. Much of this section uses Wadler, G.I. & Hainline, B. "Drugs and the Athlete", Philadelphia, F.A. Davis and Co. (1989).
2. Goldman, B., op. cit. p. 47 (1992).
3. Voy, R. (1991), op. cit.
4. Australia, "Drugs in Sport", Interim Report of the Senate Standing Committee on the Environment, Recreation and the Arts, Canberra, Australian Government Publishing Service (1989).

Initially the use of the drug was confined to the power disciplines such as weight lifting and the throwing events, but its use soon spread to swimmers and, in the United States, to football players, leading the Czech, and later American, Olympic Gold medal winning athlete and coach Olga Fikotova-Connolly to comment that "there is no way in the world a woman nowadays, in the throwing events (....) can break the record unless she is on steroids. These awful drugs have changed the complexion of track and field".[1]

Use of anabolic steroids continued to be a persistent problem among elite sportsmen and women at least until 1976 when the first reliable tests for the presence of the substance in urine was developed by Manfred Donike. Tests were conducted for steroids at the Montreal Olympic Games where eleven athletes were disqualified, of which eight were disqualified for the use of anabolic steroids. However, this landmark in the battle to eradicate steroid use represented simply the first stage in a continuing campaign. Not surprisingly, reliable epidemiological evidence about steroid use is in short supply. A survey, conducted in the early 1970s, of male Swedish elite track and field athletes concluded that 31% had used anabolic steroids.[2] Data from the United States collected in the 1980s suggested that use among college athletes was between 15% to 20%, with football players being among the heaviest users.[3] In addition, there has been a steady stream of anecdotal evidence of continuing use among athletes across a wide range of sports.

The 1980 Moscow Olympic Games were dubbed the "Junkie Olympics" by one observer who commented that "There is hardly a medal winner at the Moscow games, certainly not a gold medal winner, who is not on one sort of drug or another: usually several kinds. The Moscow games might as well have been called the Chemists' games.".[4] The allegations of extensive drug use at the Moscow games contrast with the lack of any positive test results. According to some observers the Soviet's secret service, the KGB, ensured that no drug scandals would cloud the Soviet organisational triumph.[5] However, when the samples collected at Moscow were re-analysed by Professor Manfred Donike, a senior member of the IOC Medical Commission, he found evidence of a large number of athletes using steroids.

By far the most serious scandal of the early 1980s occurred at the 1983 Pan-American Games held in Caracas, Venezuela, when not only did many athletes withdraw from the games when they were informed of the new and

1. Quoted in Goldman, B., op. cit. (1992).
2. Ljungqvist, A. "The Use of Anabolic Steroids in Top Swedish Athletes", *British Journal of Sports Medicine*, Vol. 9.2, (1975).
3. Dezelsky, T.L., Toohey, J.V. and Shaw, R.S. "Non-medical Drug Use Behavior at Five United States Universities, A Fifteen-Year Study", *Bulletin of Narcotics*, Vol. 37. P. 49, (1985); Pope et al, op. cit. (1988).
4. Australia (1989), op. cit. p. 10.
5. Jennings, A. "The New Lords of the Rings", Simon and Schuster, (1996), p. 235.

more rigorous drug-testing regime in place, but nineteen athletes from ten countries including the United States and Canada tested positive for drugs, mainly steroids. In May 1987, thirty-four people, including the British Olympic medalist David Jenkins, were indicted by United States drug enforcement agencies on 110 counts relating to conspiracy to manufacture, smuggle and distribute huge quantities of anabolic steroids. The following year the positive test on the Canadian sprinter Ben Johnson shocked the sporting world. Johnson's breath-taking run in the 100 metres race made him an immediate international hero. He was lauded in the Canadian and world press as an exceptionally gifted athlete, a perception which was transformed overnight as a result of the announcement of the positive test for the anabolic steroid stanozolol.

By the late 1980s the use of anabolic steroids had become so widespread that one estimate suggested that of all the positive results at the eighteen IOC accredited laboratories throughout the world, 70% were for anabolic steroids.[1] More recently, a survey of developments in research into the effects of steroids in the first half of the 1990s reported a series of cases demonstrating the extent to which steroid use is deeply rooted in elite sport. Among the cases reported was that of a 14-year-old South African female runner who tested positive, making her probably the youngest athlete to be caught using steroids, and the banning of a paralympic athlete for steroid use.[2] In a study of body builders in the Flanders region of Belgium, between 38% and 58% of those tested had used steroids between 1988 and 1993.[3] A total of 11% of high school football players in Arkansas high schools were also reported to be taking anabolic steroids.[4]

Although the late 1980s may have marked the high point of steroid use, the decline in the number of positives was less likely the result of more intensive testing and greater vigilance in the wake of the Johnson scandal than the fact that drug-using athletes were moving on to other more sophisticated drugs such as human growth hormone (hGH) and recombinant erythropoietin (rEPO), both of which are impossible to detect. Nevertheless, use of anabolic steroids continued into the 1990s with a number of high profile athletes testing positive including Harry "Butch" Reynolds and Randy Barnes, both American record holders in track and field sports. In Europe, in 1992, the German sprinter Katrin Krabbe tested positive for the anabolic agent clenbuterol.

1. Australia, op. cit. p. 26 (1989).
2. Bahrke, M.S., Yesalis, C.E. & Wright, J.E, "Psychological and Behavioural Effects of Endogenous Testosterone and Anabolic-Androgenic Steroids, An Update", Sports Medicine, Vol. 22.6, pp. 367- 390 (1996).
3. Delbeke, F., Desmet, N. & Debackere, "The Abuse of Doping Agents in Competing Body Builders in Flanders (1988-1993)", International Journal of Sports Medicine, Vol. 16.1, pp. 66-70 (1995).
4. Herrmann, M., "Steroids, A Vague Threat", Newsday, 30 Oct. (1988).

Cocaine

Of all the drugs used in substantial quantities by modern athletes, cocaine has probably the longest history. The stimulant and anorexiant properties of the leaves of the coca bush, a plant indigenous to Peru, were well known long before the arrival of the European invaders. Among the Incas, coca leaves were regularly used when travelling long distances to increase energy and endurance, and also to reduce hunger. Indeed "distances were measured by the number of doses of coca leaf needed in a day's travel".[1] By the time of Pizarro's conquest of Peru on behalf of Spain in the 1530s, abuse of the drug had become uncontrolled and widespread.[2] The properties of the coca leaf were swiftly reported to Europe and scientific analysis of the plants brought back was soon under way. However, it was not until the middle of the nineteenth century that scientists were successful in isolating the alkaloid cocaine from the coca leaf. As with both steroids and amphetamines, it was war that created the stimulus for more extensive experimentation with the effects of the drug on human physiology. In the 1880s the drug was administered to Bavarian troops by the army physician, Ashenbrandt, as a method of delaying the onset of fatigue.

By the early part of the present century the use of cocaine was widespread, largely as a result of being heavily promoted by Freud in Europe and Halstead in the United States. The drug was claimed to possess qualities that were beneficial in the treatment of a broad range of ailments including cancer and, ironically, morphine and alcohol addiction. Angelo Mariani developed a very popular drink produced by combining two ounces of coca leaf with one pint of wine. So popular was his mixture that it received testimonials from three popes, sixteen heads of state, and 8000 physicians.[3] Most famously the coca leaf was one of the original ingredients in the soft drink, Coca Cola, invented by John Smythe Pemberton in 1886. It was only in 1906 that the company agreed to alter the recipe and find an alternative to the coca leaf.

The emergence of the current problem with the illegal social use of cocaine began in the 1960s, developing first in the United States but spreading quickly to Europe. It is at about the same time that reports of cocaine use among sportsmen began to surface, especially among football players in the United States. The first of a continuing series of deaths associated with cocaine use among athletes occurred in the early 1980s. The death, in 1980, of Terry Furlow (basketball) was followed by Billy Ylvisaker (polo) in 1983, but it was the trio of deaths in 1986 in the United States that drew the attention of sports organisations and the public to the extent and seriousness of cocaine abuse among athletes. In 1986 Larry Gordon (football), Don Rogers

---

1. Kunkel, D.B., "Cocaine then and now. Part I, Its History, Medical Botany, and Use", *Emergency Medicine*, June 15th (1986).
2. Walder, G.I. & Hainline, B., op. cit. (1989), p. 87.
3. Kunkel, D.B. p.128 (1986), op. cit.

(also football) and the bright basketball prospect, Len Bias, all died.[1] By 1986 there was substantial evidence of extensive use among college and professional athletes. A 1984 survey of over 2000 NCAA athletes reported that 13% were currently taking cocaine with a total of 17% admitting using cocaine in the previous twelve months.[2] These findings were supported by a later survey of elite women athletes which found that 7% of respondents acknowledged using cocaine.[3]

Human growth hormone

Human growth hormone (hGH) is one of the newest drugs to be exploited for competitive advantage by athletes. hGH was developed in the mid 1980s as a replacement for natural growth hormone extracted from the pituitary glands of cadavers when the latter was deemed unsafe because of the possibility of the transmission of infections, such as Creutzfeldt-Jakob disease (CJD). Because the range of medical conditions for which hGH is used is small the amount commercially produced is still limited, thus restricting its availability for illicit use by athletes.[4] However, since the development of synthetic hGH there has been a large number of enquiries about the drug from athletes.[5] In 1983 it was revealed that athletes competing in Helsinki had been using hGH. Although none of the 200 samples taken tested positive, traces of hGH were found in some of the samples when retested at the IOC accredited laboratory at Cologne.[6] By the late 1980s there had already been cases of athletes reputedly using hGH at twenty times the normal level and one case of a doctor attempting to buy large amounts of the drug and selling it for non-medical purposes.[7]

One of the few recorded examples of misuse of the drug by an athlete was uncovered during the enquiries made at the time of Justice Dubin's investigation of drug abuse by Canadian athletes following the Ben Johnson scandal. During the hearings the Canadian sprinter, Angella Issajenko, admitted using hGH along with other drugs. According to the Dubin Report, the fact that the drug is tightly controlled has not prevented it becoming available to athletes. Notwithstanding the strict control of growth hormone, there was evidence of increased use by other sprinters, body builders, weightlifters, and intercollegiate football players whose sole source of supply has been the black market.[8] The attraction of hGH to athletes is not just that it is thought

---

1. Voy, R. (1991), op. cit., p. 8.
2. Anderson, W.A. & McKeag, D.B. (1985). A survey by Michigan State University College of Human Medicine, 1984.
3. Elite Women Athletic Survey. Hazelden Health Promotion Services, Minneapolis (1987).
4. According to the Dubin Report there is only one legitimate medical use for hGH.
5. Wadler, G.I. & Hainline, B. (1989), op. cit.; Cowart, V.S. "Human Growth Hormone, The Latest Ergogenic Aid", Physician and Sports Medicine, Vol. 16.3 (1988).
6. Donohoe, T. & Johnson, N., p. 113 (1986), op. cit.
7. Cowart, V.S., op. cit. (1988).
8. Dubin Inquiry, Commission of Inquiry into the Use of Drugs and Banned Practices Intended to Increase Athletic Performance, Commissioner, Charles L. Dubin, Ottawa, Canadian Government Printing Centre, p. 120 (1990).

by many athletes to produce an effect similar to anabolic steroids but, more importantly, that it is currently undetectable. The drug seems to be less attractive to those seeking to build muscle strength and more attractive to those, such as body builders, seeking to improve musculature and a more sculpted effect.[1]

Evidence of the use of the drug has also been found among adolescents who may take the drug for sport-related purposes such as attempting to ensure sufficient growth for height-related sports. Evidence of abuse has also been found among those adolescents seeking to improve their physique simply for cosmetic purposes.[2]

Diuretics

Diuretics are drugs that are used to increase the rate of urine formation. In sport they are used to achieve rapid weight loss in weight-related sports such as wrestling, judo, weight-lifting and boxing. They can also be used to flush out other drugs, thus making detection more difficult. A third use of diuretics is to overcome the side effect of fluid retention resulting from the use of androgenic anabolic steroids. The use of diuretics in conjunction with this class of steroids helps body builders in particular to achieve a more sharply defined musculature or "cut look".[3]

Positive tests for diuretics occasionally occur, and one of the first cases involved a Canadian athlete who, in order to make his weight category for an event in Caracas in 1983 "ran outside at noon in two jogging suits, covered with plastic garbage bags, with a hat, trying to sweat off as much weight as he could, as much water as he could and, at the same time, was using diuretics". Not surprisingly the athlete collapsed.[4] No breach of doping regulations had taken place because diuretics were not, at that time, on the IOC list of banned substances, although they were added in 1985. Since the inclusion of diuretics on the IOC list there have been a small but regular number of positive results. One of the most serious examples of the abuse of diuretics occurred at the Seoul Olympics where the British athlete Kerrith Brown won a bronze medal in the judo competition but later tested positive for the diuretic frusemide. In the same year, during the 1988 Tour de France, Pedro Delgado tested positive for diuretics which he was using as a masking agent. The scandal was exacerbated by the response of the French newspaper *Le Monde* which claimed that the international authorities, in monitoring for drugs, had "broken the heart" of the Tour de France.

---

1. George, A. "The Anabolic steroids and Peptide Hormones", in Mottram, D.R. (1996), op. cit., p. 208.
2. Ibid , p. 209.
3. Verroken, M. "Drug use and Abuse in Sport", in Mottram, D. R., op. cit., p. 35 (1996).
4. Remarks of Dr Pipe, quoted in Australia (1989), op. cit. p. 117.

The impact of doping on sport: the example of swimming

A study in the mid 1980s states that there was little evidence regarding the particular drugs favoured by swimmers but suggested that there were five categories of drugs in common use by swimmers and other athletes involved in aquatic sports, namely anabolic steroids, psychomotor stimulants, sympathomimetic amines, non-steroidal inflammatory drugs, and recreational (social) drugs.[1] The range of drugs attractive to aquatic athletes is broadly the same as those used by the majority of track and field abusers. What distinguishes swimming from other sports is the seriousness of the doping infractions, their persistence and the impact on the sport.

Two episodes are worthy of mention: the first concerns the dominance of Olympic and world championship swimming by the East Germans in the 1970s and 1980s and the second concerns the much more recent domination of swimming by athletes from the People's Republic of China. In the 1970s, many of the rumours of drug abuse that surrounded the outstanding success of the swimmers from the GDR were rejected as the product of envy rather than evidence. However, evidence soon began to accumulate, first through the testimony of defectors and later from documentary sources following the ending of the cold war. In 1979, for example, Renate Vogel, the 1974 100-metre breaststroke world record holder, defected to the West and recounted stories of systematic use of anabolic steroids. Later evidence cast doubt over many medal winning and record-breaking performances by the East Germans and posed a serious problem for the international federation in deciding how to deal with artificially high world records.

The dilemma was compounded in the early 1990s by the remarkable emergence of swimmers from the People's Republic of China (PRC). At the 1988 Olympics the PRC women's team collected only four medals, none of which was gold. Six years later, at the Rome World Championships, the PRC team collected a startling twelve gold medals out of a possible sixteen events. At the time some commentators drew attention to the masculine physique of many of the female swimmers, the rapidity of improvement, the fact that the PRC swimmers were dominating in the power events (freestyle and butterfly, rather than the disciplines requiring greater technical sophistication) and the presence in China of coaches from the former East Germany from 1988 to 1990. A further cause of suspicion was the fact that the dramatic improvement was almost completely confined to the female squad despite the declaration by the Chinese that male and females trained as an integrated squad with a similar training regime. These suspicions led to accusations from the Chinese of racism and jealousy on the part of the critics, but scientific confirmation was quick to emerge.

---

1. Puffer, J.C. "The Use of Drugs in Swimming", *Clinics in Sports Medicine*, Vol. 5.1, (1986).

Four positive tests were recorded around the time of the Rome World Championships, seven a month later at the Asian Games and eight more to follow by March 1995; all but one of the positive test results were for steroids. As Carlile recounts, the evidence was only provided as a result of the application of extremely sophisticated analytic testing methods involving the development by a Japanese laboratory of a method of detecting the presence of dihydrotestosterone (DHT), "a sophisticated, endogenously produced hormone like testosterone – though much more potent and with a faster clearance time".[1] Following the Rome competition and two weeks before the Chinese squad left for the Asian Games, out-of-competition tests were conducted on two swimmers. The results were positive although the results were not made public immediately. Two weeks later, when the Chinese team arrived in Hiroshima three days before the start of competition, a number of swimmers were selected for immediate testing and five more provided positive results with persistent rumours that another seven or more results were borderline. By testing the members of the Chinese team so early, the sampling officers increased the probability of catching those who had tried to cut their clearance period too fine.

The scale of drug abuse by the Chinese is not the only or even the most significant aspect of this episode. Of greater significance is the attitude of the IOC on the one hand and the President of the Chinese Olympic Committee on the other. The IOC was clearly aware of the scale of doping taking place in China in the early 1990s but chose not to inform FINA, the international federation for swimming, of the number of positive results reported to the Chinese authorities. In addition, the president of the IOC, Juan Samaranch, stated "I do not think the Chinese are using drugs" only to be contradicted by Manfred Donike, a leading authority on doping, who stated "There is systematic doping with the substance DHT".[2] Of greater concern was the attitude of the president of the Chinese Olympic Committee who stated that "we will not have foreigners coming into China as investigators, closely examining our sports preparations in such a systematic and probing way".[3]

The spate of positive test results and the mounting evidence of state collusion in systematic doping provoked an outcry among other members of the Olympic movement, not only because of the scale of the cheating but also due to a mounting sense of frustration at the apparent inability or reluctance of the IOC and FINA to pull China into line. There was much talk of banning China from participation from all swimming events until it could prove that its athletes were drug free. In addition, there was understandable anger among the number of swimmers who were, in all probability, denied a medal

---

1. Carlile, F. "Why the Chinese must not swim at Atlanta ' 96", *Inside Sport*, November, pp. 18-29, (1995).
2. Ibid.,
3. Ibid.,

because of the actions of the Chinese. Finally, the international federation is left with the problem of artificially inflated world record times. Given the importance of record-breaking in selling events to the media, inflated records not only defraud legitimate athletes but make a sport less attractive to the much-needed sponsors.

Hopes that the issue of Chinese doping had ended with the furore that followed the Rome World Championships were proved unfounded when a series of equally serious incidents occurred at the World Championships held in Perth in 1998. On arrival, one swimmer was found to be carrying a flask containing thirteen glass vials of human growth hormone, enough, according to the FINA secretary, to supply the whole squad. The drug seizure was followed by four positive test results on other members of the squad. The net effect was to overshadow the championships and add fuel to the suspicion that systematic doping was taking place in China. Such was the seriousness of the episode that IOC President, Juan Samaranch, commented that the incident had indeed harmed any plans that China might have of bidding for the 2008 Olympic Games.

Conclusion

Although the sophistication and, possibly, the extent of drug use by athletes is the product of the last forty years or so, doping has been associated with competitive sport for far longer. In the eighteenth and nineteenth centuries the major commercial and professional sports, including boxing, cycling and running, all provided ample evidence of substantial drug use. Commercialisation must be considered an important element in any discussion of contemporary doping. A further consideration must be the development of scientific capacity to synthesise drugs in the early and middle part of the present century. The dramatic advances made by the pharmaceutical industry enabled athletes to substitute safer drugs for the more dangerous and to select drugs tailored to meet the requirements of particular sports or training regimes.

The advances by the pharmaceutical industry were also given added momentum by the second world war and the blurring of peacetime morality with the expediency of wartime. Wartime not only added urgency to the search for new drugs which would be beneficial to troops but, much more importantly, also changed the moral climate regarding drug use. Wartime was a period during which governments sanctioned and organised drug use by soldiers. The moral ambiguity surrounding the use of drugs in wartime continued into the cold war period and entered the Olympic arena as sport emerged, along with space, as surrogates for military conflict. The power of cold war politics to affect the judgement of those who cared deeply about sport is amply illustrated by the actions of Dr Ziegler discussed above in connection with the use of steroids by the American team.

A further complicating factor in the spread of doping in contemporary society is the blurred boundary between social/recreational drug use and drug use for competitive advantage. In attempting to define an appropriate policy response to doping in sport, it is not possible to target either athletes or specific drugs which are unique to sport. Athletes, like everyone else, get ill and have a social life and doping authorities have considerable difficulties in dealing with proprietary medicines and remedies for chronic complaints such as asthma. There are also problems in responding to positive test results for drugs with no proven ergogenic property such as cannabis. In addition, attempts to focus the policy response on particular types of drugs also has pitfalls as many drugs favoured by athletes are also used socially or for non-sporting purposes. The abuse of amphetamines, cocaine and, more recently, anabolic steroids is not limited to athletes, thus multiplying the sources of supply and the consequent problems of control.

The involvement of Dr Ziegler in the promotion of steroids in the United States not only draws attention to the significance of the cold war in affecting moral judgement but also to the central role of medical doctors in the spread of drug use. Dr Ziegler, who, once he realised the destructive potential of steroids for sport as well as individual athletes campaigned for the rest of his life against doping in sport, was the first of a series of doctors involved in facilitating drug use in sport. Ben Johnson's doping regime was carefully prepared and monitored by his doctor, Jamie Astaphan, who "had been heavily involved for many years in the planning, supervision, and administration of steroid programs for many athletes".[1] In the United States, Dr Robert Kerr estimated that in the mid 1980s there were at least seventy physicians in the Los Angeles area who prescribed anabolic steroids to athletes. He himself has prescribed them for athletes from the United States, Canada, South America, Australia and the Far East.[2] Dr Ara Artinian of Toronto who dealt mainly with football players and body builders prescribed over US$ 200000 of steroids between 1981 and 1988. The Black committee of the Australian Senate heard that 41% of body builders in Australia obtained their supply of steroids from doctors.[3]

The depth of involvement of doctors is especially worrying as one would expect the medical profession to adhere to a morality that would exclude such behaviour. Yet doctors are only the most prominent in a long list of professionals in positions of trust who have systematically abused that trust by encouraging, colluding, or at best ignoring the continuing use of steroids. Pharmacists, coaches and officials are all implicated in the steady increase in drug abuse in sport. Given the range of sports professionals involved in

---

1. Dubin Inquiry, p. 285, op. cit. (1990).
2. Ibid, p. 357.
3. Ibid, p. 357.

doping, the question arises of the position of athletes and their degree of culpability. Although many drug-abusing athletes are responsible for initiating and controlling their use of drugs, there are many who, either through intimidation or ignorance, are arguably less responsible. Should we always assume that the athlete is the villain rather than the victim? This question is especially important when the application of penalties is considered. While athletes are the focus for disciplinary action, it is still comparatively rare for the coaches and managers who condoned the use of drugs, the doctors who prescribed the drugs, and the pharmacists who supplied the drugs to face any significant penalties.[1]

The development of an effective policy response to doping depends on an ability to identify accurately all those involved in the supply, distribution, encouragement and use of drugs whether they are individual sportsmen and women or sports and government organisations. There is a danger that athletes are being targeted not just because they are guilty of abusing drugs but also because they are one of the easier targets in what is a much more complex and widespread pattern of culpability.

---

1. This issue is discussed in Chapter 8.

Chapter 3

Banned substances and practices and their effects

The drugs used by athletes in the nineteenth century and earlier were derived mainly from plants, animals or microbiological sources. From plants came drugs such as cocaine, morphine and digitalis; from animals came steroids; and from microbiology came penicillin and streptomycin, all of which contributed significant advances in the treatment of ailments but which also provided a number of drugs which could be used in the attempt to gain an advantage in competition, such as the chewing of coca leaves or the ingesting of sheep's testicles. The mid twentieth century marked a dramatic increase in the synthesis of drugs from plants and animals and was also the golden age in the development of anti-bacterial drugs from microbial sources.

The mid to late twentieth century has been a period of intense development and expansion in the pharmaceutical industry as chemists sought and continue to seek to identify and synthesise new drugs and refine existing products. One of the many problems facing anti-doping organisations is attempting to keep in step with the pace of pharmaceutical advance. The IOC remains in the forefront of the co-ordination and direction of the global anti-doping effort. One of the initial, but increasingly complex, problems facing the IOC is the compilation and updating of the list of banned substances and practices. Although there are signs that a number of international federations are refining or tailoring the IOC list to suit the particular characteristics of their own sport, the IOC list remains the most authoritative statement of policy. Two problems facing the IOC in compiling its list are the difficulties in determining whether a drug contravenes "the ethics of sport and medical science" and the timing of the addition of new drugs to the IOC list.

The first problem may be illustrated by comparing a definition of drugs given by Mottram with the definition of doping provided by the IOC. For Mottram, drugs "are chemical substances which, by interaction with biological targets, can alter the biochemical systems of the body".[1] His definition is an objective statement, quite properly devoid of any normative aspect. However, he does add a reminder that "drugs are designed to rectify imbalances of biochemical systems which have been induced by disease. They are not primarily designed to affect biochemical systems in healthy subjects".[2] The IOC's

---

1. Mottram, D.R. "Drugs in Sport" (2nd edn.) London, E & FN Spon (1996), p. 1.
2. Ibid, p.1.

definition of doping is an extension of Mottram's caveat and states that: "Doping contravenes the ethics of both sport and medical science. Doping consists of: the administration of substances belonging to prohibited classes of pharmacological agents, and/or the use of various prohibited methods".[1]

The IOC is shrewd in dividing the policy statement into two discrete sentences, the first of which states the committee's moral position on doping while the second is a simple statement of the categories of activity that contravene IOC rules. Although the two statements are linked, it is clear that the second does not (legally at least) depend on the first. In the elaboration of its policy statement the IOC identifies three categories of prohibited substances or actions: doping classes, doping methods and classes of drugs subject to certain restrictions. The category of doping classes includes stimulants, narcotic analgesics, anabolic agents, diuretics, and peptide and glycoprotein hormones and analogues. Doping methods covers blood doping and pharmacological, chemical and physical manipulation. The final category, classes of drugs subject to certain restrictions, refers to alcohol, marijuana, local anaesthetics, corticosteroids and beta-blockers. See Appendix A for the complete IOC list of banned substances and practices.

Stimulants

The list of stimulants is considerable and covers those substances designed to achieve some or all of the following: increased alertness, reduced fatigue and increased competitiveness and aggression. Among the most commonly abused stimulants in sport are amphetamines, cocaine, caffeine and other sympathomimetic amines such as ephedrine.

Amphetamines

The category of drugs referred to as stimulants function by stimulating the body's central nervous system. The first stimulants to be used extensively in sport in the post-war period were amphetamines which are attractive to athletes because they mimic physiological changes in the body that occur at times of stress and danger. The body's normal response to stress and danger is often referred to as "fight or flight". In these situations the body's sympathetic nervous system is activated and the changes that occur include an increased flow of blood through the muscles, and an increase in concentration and alertness. In these processes the release of epinephrine by the adrenal glands plays a significant role and drugs that act in a similar manner are called sympathomimetic.[2] Amphetamine is closely related in structure to

---

1. IOC Medical Commission "Prohibited Classes of Substances and Prohibited Methods", Lausanne, IOC (6th November 1996).
2. Strauss, R.H., "Drugs in Sports", in Strauss, R.H. (ed.), *Sports Medicine*, Philadelphia, W.B. Saunders (1984), p. 485.

epinephrine and stimulates the central nervous system to release neurotrans-mitters from the nerve terminals.

Amphetamine has proved attractive to athletes for a variety of reasons and across a wide range of sports. For some the attraction lies in the capacity of the drug to provide an artificial way to prepare psychologically for competition. This use is most common in sports where aggression is an important element, such as in contact sports including American football, ice hockey and rugby, and in explosive sports such as the shot, weightlifting and hammer. Amphetamines are also used in some endurance sports which require sustained consumption of energy, such as cycling, running and swimming. Finally, amphetamines are also used in some weight-graded sports to suppress appetite in order to facilitate weight loss.

In attempting to assess the value of drugs in enhancing performance, the primary stumbling block is the lack of valid double-blind experimental data. Much of the "evidence" for the ergogenic effects of amphetamines is anecdotal rather than scientific. A rare, scientifically valid study concluded that the use of amphetamines produced a small improvement in swimming (0.59% to 1.16%), running (1.5%) and weight-throwing (3% to 4%).[1] However, even this study was criticised for failing to control variables adequately and there must consequently be concern at the validity of the conclusions.[2] The researchers also focused on a narrow range of skills applied in sport; skills of note in other sports such as hand-eye co-ordination, judgement, timing and steadiness of hand were not evaluated.

Some supporting evidence for the ergogenic value of amphetamines is available from studies on animals which have shown increased endurance in swimming and running.[3] A survey of existing evidence suggested that amphetamine use can improve performance but that the margin of improvement was only of a few percent.[4] However, the authors were acutely aware of the significance of that apparently disappointing conclusion as they noted that among elite athletes a few percentage points may mean the difference between first and fourth. More significantly, they conclude that there was "an amphetamine margin" and that "amphetamines can confer a significant competitive edge in sports. (...) Moreover their versatility is so remarkable that they enhance acute bursts of strength as well as the ability to cope with prolonged challenges to endurance".[5] Most tellingly they point out that in

---

1. Smith, G.M. & Beecher, H.K., "Amphetamine sulphate and Athletic Performance", *Journal of the American Medical Association*, 170 (1959).
2. George, A., op. cit., p. 91 (1996).
3. Bhagat, B. & Wheeler, N., "Effect of Amphetamines on the Swimming Endurance of Rats", *Neuropharmacology*, Vol. 12, (1973); Gerald, M.C. "Effects of (+)-amphetamine on the Treadmill Performance of Rats", *Neuropharmacology*, Vol. 17, pp.703-704 (1978).
4. Laties, V.G. & Weiss, B., "The Amphetamine Margin in Sports", *Federation of the American Society for Experimental Biology*, Vol. 40.12 (1981).
5. Ibid., p. 2691.

the one-mile race there had only been a 15% improvement in the world record in the 100 years up to 1975 and that it therefore takes between six and seven years to produce a 1% improvement. As a result, anyone who was able to improve a near world record time by 1% would be able to create a world record that would take many years to better.

Other experiments have suggested a much more variable impact of amphetamine use. One showed an improvement in three in twenty athletes and also found a reduction in performance in one in twenty.[1] It would appear that while improved performance is indeed possible, the effect is not uniform across all athletes and, equally importantly, is not uniform across all sports or roles within team sports. One study found that, while amphetamine use improved some aspects of athletic performance, it did not result in improved sprinting.[2] Another study of the use of amphetamines, this time of American football players, found that linesmen often used high doses of the drug but that the effect was negative insofar as linesmen were often less able to adjust their game to changes in team tactics, frequently being unaware that they were repeating the same positional plays.[3]

Leaving aside the question of the possible benefits to sporting performance, it must be borne in mind that a completely non-toxic drug does not exist.[4] The side effects of amphetamines are substantial, with loss of judgement and the development of dependence being the most significant. Indeed, many athletes who have used amphetamines think they have performed much better than they have in reality. Amphetamines engender a mood of heightened optimism which interferes with judgement.[5] A diminution of judgement in endurance races is potentially very dangerous as the athlete may exceed his or her physical limits just as the cyclist Tom Simpson did during the Tour de France. Research has confirmed that the use of amphetamines by cyclists impaired their ability to recognise that they were exceeding their toleration of exertion and heat and thus may explain the high incidence of cardiac problems and heatstroke in the sport.[6] A similar loss of judgement was found among American football players taking amphetamines who often continued playing after injury and often in considerable pain.[7] Further, an athlete's loss of judgement in a contact sport may result in the unnecessary injury of others through overly aggressive play.

---

1. Karpovich, P.V., "Effects of amphetamine sulphate on athletic performance", Journal of the American Medical Association, 170 (1959).
2. Chandler, J.V. & Blair, S.N., "The Effects of Amphetamines on Selected Physiological Components Related to Athletic Success", Med. Sci. Sports Exercise, Vol. 12, pp. 65-69 (1980).
3. Mandell, A.J., Stewart, K.D. & Russo, P.V. "The Sundat Syndrome, From Kinetics to Altered Consciousness", Federation of the American Society for Experimental Biology, Vol. 40.12 (1981).
4. Mottram, D.R., op. cit. (1996) p. 10.
5. Strauss, R.H (1984), op. cit.
6. Wyndham, G.H., Roger, G.G., Benade, A.J.S. & Strydan, N.B. "Physiological Effects of Amphetamines during Exercise", South African Medical Journal, Vol. 45, pp. 247-52 (1971).
7. Mandell, A.J., "The Nightmare Season" New York, Random House (1976).

It has also been reported that tolerance of amphetamines develops rapidly leading to a situation where as much as one gram of amphetamine was required by established users to produce the same effects as ten milligrams to thirty milligrams had on new users. Dependence may also lead to psychotic aggression and withdrawal is associated with mental and physical depression.[1] In addition, amphetamine use has also been known to cause paranoia, anorexia, insomnia, hypertension, cardiac arrhythmias and tremor. The scientific evidence regarding the benefits to athletes of amphetamines is variable and ambiguous. Where amphetamines do have a perceived benefit in some sports or team positions, it may well be that the effect is more psychological than physiological.

Cocaine

Many of the comments made about the properties of amphetamines apply to other major stimulants. Cocaine was, in many respects, the precursor of amphetamine and its history of enthusiastic embrace by the medical profession followed by a steady decline in prescription and a growing awareness of the serious side effects of the drug broadly anticipated that of amphetamine. Like amphetamine, cocaine operates by affecting the central nervous system and has a powerful effect on mood. Cocaine appears to operate in part through the non-thinking part of the brain which governs reflexes and which serves emotional, sexual drive and memory functions. "It is the pharmacological manipulation of the 'pleasure brain' that explains neurologically the compulsivity, preoccupation, craving and relapse behavior so often seen in cocaine users".[2] Although both amphetamine and cocaine create dependence, it is the power of cocaine's addictive properties that distinguishes it from amphetamine. Apart from providing a short-term feeling of euphoria (estimated to be between ten minutes to three hours depending on method of administration and the extent of habituation), cocaine has a mild local anaesthetic effect but also raises blood pressure.

Being specific about the physiological effects of cocaine is extremely difficult as there are few reliable scientific studies and much of the qualitative data is anecdotal and, more importantly, based on the consumption of cocaine that is rarely free of impurities. Cocaine, sold illegally, is frequently adulterated with other stimulants such as caffeine and phenylpropanolamine, local anaesthetics such as procaine, hallucinogens such as LSD, depressants such as diazepam, and other less expensive substances designed to dilute the drug such as talcum powder, sucrose and sodium bicarbonate.

It has been claimed that "this powerful stimulant can produce feelings of euphoria and is capable of improving some aspects of performance through

---

1. George is referring to research undertaken by Brookes and reported in George, A. "Central Nervous System Stimulants", in Mottram, D.R., op. cit. (1996).
2. Wadler, G.I. & Hainline, B. p. 90, op. cit. (1989).

61

prolonged endurance".[1] However, it is impossible to draw valid conclusions about the effect of cocaine on athletic performance. The absence of scientific data notwithstanding, there is a perception among athletes that cocaine does possess ergogenic properties.[2] One of the very few scientific studies was carried out by Freud over 100 years ago from which he concluded that intranasal cocaine increased muscle strength for up to three hours: however, this conclusion has been contradicted by more recent research[3] which is far from conclusive. Such evidence available prior to 1983 has been poorly designed and generally unreliable.[4]

In practice most, admittedly subjective, assessments suggest that cocaine use results in a deterioration in athletic performance. Hand-eye co-ordination, general concentration and deterioration in team discipline are all considered to be consequences of cocaine use.[5] However, the anecdotal evidence, particularly from within football in North America, indicates that the growth in cocaine use among athletes has been for recreational rather than ergogenic motives.

The side effects of cocaine abuse are serious and are not simply limited to the creation of a level of dependence that led one researcher to refer to cocaine as "possibly the most addictive agent known".[6] The list of adverse side effects of cocaine use is both long and daunting, including cardiac and neuropsychiatric problems. Cardiac problems include strokes (rupture of the brain's blood vessels) and myocardial infarction: neuropsychiatric problems include paranoia, psychosis, repetitive behaviour and anorexia. The danger of cocaine use is indicated by the increased incidence of sudden deaths among users. One hypothesis is that athletes may be especially susceptible to a fatal reaction to cocaine as a dose of the drug large enough to produce a seizure combined with their muscle composition may result in a lethal production of heat and lactic acid causing cardiac failure.[7]

Caffeine

Caffeine is also included in the stimulant category and is subject to IOC restrictions. The "physiological effects of caffeine include diuresis, gastric

---

1. Donohoe, T & Johnson, N., *Foul Play, Drug Abuse in Sports*, Oxford, Blackwell (1986).
2. Puffer, J., "The Use of Drugs in Swimming", *Clinics in Sports Medicine*, Vol. 5, pp.77-89, (1986).
3. Ritchie, J.M. & Green, N.M. "Local anesthetics" in Gillman, A.G. et al (eds) *Goodman and Gillman's the Pharmacological Basis of Therapeutics*, (7th edn.) New York, Macmillan (1985).
4. Conlee, R.K., "Amphetamine, Caffeine and Cocaine" in *Perspectives in Exercise Science and Sports Medicine*, Lamb, D.R. & Williams, M.H. (eds.), New York, Brown & Benchmark (1991), see also Haddad, L.M. "Cocaine Abuse, Background, Clinical Presentation, and Emergency Treatment", *Internal Medicine for the Specialist*, Vol.7.9, pp. 67-75 (1986).
5. Ibid, p. 96.
6. George, A., op. cit., p. 97.
7. Giammarco, R.A., "The Athlete, Cocaine and Lactic Acidosis, a Hypothesis", *American Journal of Medical Sciences*, Vol. 294, pp. 412-414, (1987).

acid release, smooth muscle relaxation, increased contractility of skeletal muscle, increased lipolysis, and increased heart rate, blood pressure, oxygen consumption and metabolic rate".[1] In addition to the metabolic benefits of caffeine, the specific competitive benefit of caffeine might also be due to its capacity to stimulate the central nervous system.[2]

The current IOC restriction on the use of caffeine identifies the threshold for a doping infraction to be 12 micrograms per millilitre (about four to eight cups of coffee in a period of two or three hours). Caffeine, as an ergogenic aid, is claimed to increase endurance, and to result in heightened alertness and improved concentration, but the effect varies according to dosage and sport, and scientific opinion is far from a consensus. Even with the ingestion of doses below the IOC threshold there is a discernible, though extremely slight effect on athletes involved in short duration high-performance events, but the effect of larger doses in endurance events and in some short-term high intensity sports is defined as significant.[3] Supporting evidence suggests that work output can increase up to 7% and the duration of exercise time can increase by 19%.[4] In addition, the administration of modest amounts of caffeine (equivalent to two and a half cups of coffee) in controlled experiments has increased the endurance of athletes and non-athletes when cycling to exhaustion.[5] However, the evidence is not conclusive. A review of current research, reported that a number of studies conclude that caffeine had no ergogenic effect on muscle strength and fatigue, output, work capacity, (and) maximal swimming speed.[6] Ergogenic effects on other capacities and skills required in sport do not seem to be present: steadiness and reaction time appear to be either unaffected or adversely affected by caffeine.[7] There are many possible reasons for the contradictory nature of experimental results including the lack of standardisation in experimental conditions, the complexity of the impact of caffeine on the body, and the significance of the athlete's extent of use of caffeine prior to administration for experimental purposes. Moreover, it is possible that caffeine is of ergogenic value only in a limited number of sports and in precise conditions.[1]

1. Scwenk, T.L. "Psychoactive Drugs and Athletic Performance", *The Physician and Sports Medicine*, Vol. 25.1. pp. 33-46 (1997).

2. Rall, T.W. "Central Nervous Stimulants-the Methylxanthines" in Gillman, A.G. et al (eds), *Goodman and Gillman's the Pharmacological Basis of Therapeutics*, (7th edn.), New York, Macmillan (1985).

3. Dodd, S.L., Herb, R.A & Powers, S.K., "Caffeine and Exercise Performance", *Sports Medicine*, Vol. 15.1, pp. 4-23 (1993).

4. Graham, T.E. & Spriet L.L. "Caffeine and exercise Performance", *Sports Science Exchange*, Vol. 9, pp. 1-6 (1996).

5. Costill, D.L., Dalsky, G.P. & Fink, W.J., "Effects of Caffeine Ingestion on Metabolism and Exercise Performance", *Med. Sci. Sports Exerc*, Vol. 10, pp. 155-.58. (1978).

6. Nehlig, A & Debry, G., "Caffeine and Sports Activity, A Review", Vol. 15, pp. 215-223, op. cit. (1994).

7. Franks, H.M., Hagedorn, H., Hensley,V.A. & Starmer, G.A., "The Effect of Caffeine on Human Performance Alone and in Combination with Ethanol", *Psychopharmacologia*, Vol.45, pp. 177-181 (1975); Tarnopolsky, M.A. "Caffeine and Endurance Performance", *Sports Medicine*, Vol. 18.2, pp. 109-125 (1994).

8. Nehlig, A. & Debry, G (1994), op. cit.

Despite the legality and widespread social acceptance of caffeine, it does have some negative side effects. For the habitual user denial of access to caffeine, even for a short period of a day, can result in the development of withdrawal symptoms such as headaches, dysphoria and insomnia.[1] For the athlete seeking ergogenic advantage the side effects are relatively mild and include insomnia, gastrointestinal upset, tremor, and anxiety. The diuretic properties of caffeine make its use in endurance competitions problematic.[2] But it is only at very high doses that there is a risk of seizure and delirium.[3]

Ephedrine

Ephedrine and phenylpropanolamine are sympathomimetic amines or "look-alike" drugs because they mimic the effects of amphetamines. Their use increased substantially in the 1970s and coincided, first, with the increase in a number of countries of legal controls over amphetamines and, second, with growing concern among doctors at the serious side effects of amphetamine use. As one would expect, ephedrine affects the central nervous system in a very similar way to amphetamine. Physiologically ephedrine and phenyl-propanolamine increase blood pressure and the pulse rate: psychologically, they may produce euphoria and increased alertness.[4]

Ephedrine and similar sympathomimetic amines are widely used in competitive sport due to the widespread perception that they have ergogenic properties. It is believed that they are capable of enhancing endurance and of depressing appetite and are therefore used by athletes involved in long distance cycling, swimming and running events, and also by those involved in weigh-related or graded sports, such as judo and wrestling.

The evidence of ergogenic effect is weak. In one double-blind study of twenty-one males using ephedrine or placebo, it was concluded that ephedrine had no effect on a broad range of sports-related variables including strength, endurance, hand-eye co-ordination, speed of recovery from exercise and perception of exertion.[5] A survey of existing studies of ephedrine concluded that the results, from the admittedly small number of studies, suggested that when administered at either therapeutic or twice therapeutic doses "it appears that ephedrine is not ergogenic".[6]

The side effects of ephedrine are also similar to, but less common than, those for amphetamine and include, at the extreme, hallucinations, psychosis and

---

1. Rall (1985), op. cit.
2. Tarnopolsky, M.A. (1994), op. cit.
3. Strauss, R.H. (1984), op. cit.; Stillner, V. et al "Caffeine-induced Delirium during Prolonged Competitive Stress", American Journal of Psychiatry, Vol. 135, (1978).
4. Wadler, G.I. & Hainline, B. (1989), op. cit., p.102.
5. Sidney, K.H. & Lefcoe, W.M., "The Effects of Ephedrine on the Physiological and Psychological on Submaximal and Maximal Exercises in Man", Med. Sci. Sports, Vol. 9, (1977).
6. Clarkson, P.M. & Thompson, H.S., "Drugs and Sport, Research Findings and Limitations", Sports Medicine, Vol. 24, p. 372 (1997).

compulsive behaviour. Phenylpropanolamine has been associated with some cases of extreme hypertension, but the identification of the specific side effects of the drug are difficult as it is often taken in combination with other drugs such as caffeine or non-steroidal anti-inflammatory preparations.[1]

Narcotic analgesics

Drugs within the narcotics category include diamorphine (heroin) and methadone. From the sixteenth century to the middle of the nineteenth century, opium, from which morphine is derived, was used extensively for its hypnotic and analgesic properties. Early in the nineteenth century the German pharmacist, Sertürner, isolated and described morphine, the first of a number of alkaloids of opium which were discovered during the second half of the nineteenth century. The use of the alkaloids rapidly replaced the use of opium in medical treatment.

Narcotic analgesics act primarily on the central nervous system, depressing particular centres and causing a reduction in levels of perception of pain, fear and anxiety as well as reduced powers of concentration. By acting on opiate receptors in the brain, morphine and heroin "appear to be mimicking the effect of certain endogenous opiates, known as endorphins and enkephalins, which are thought to control pain".[2]

There is little evidence that narcotics have any ergogenic properties and they have generally been used in sport to enable athletes to continue in competition after injury and also to desensitise athletes participating in contact sports where the risk of injury is high.[3] This pattern of use also constitutes the most significant, though indirect, side effect of narcotics as the exposure to greater risk of serious injury arising from the power of the drug to raise thresholds of pain beyond the natural level enables athletes to continue to compete when injured thus putting them at risk of further injury or the compounding of the initial injury. Short-term use may result in a number of adverse effects including nausea, constipation, dysphoria and dizziness, although the intensity of the effects will depend on the dose administered.[4] There are also a number of side effects that result from extended use of narcotic analgesics, the most serious of which is the rapid production of physical dependence manifest through a number of symptoms including sweating, yawning and running eyes followed by muscular cramp, diarrhoea and vomiting, and also a psychogenic dependence where the user experiences an irresistible craving for the drug. Long-term use also leads to the depression of centres in the brain that govern the respiratory system and may, in extreme cases, result in death.

---

1. Pentel, P., "Toxicity of over-the-counter stimulants", *Journal of the American Medical Association*, Vol. 252, (1984).
2. Mottram, D.R., p. 43 (1996), op. cit.
3. Rounsaville, B. et al "Neurophysiological Functioning in Opiate Addicts", *Journal of Nervous Mental Disorders*, Vol. 170, (1982).
4. Wadler, G.I & Hainline, B., p. 156 (1989), op. cit.

Anabolic agents

Anabolic-androgenic steroids

There is much evidence of a long-held belief that the testes were the source of male characteristics and, in particular, were responsible for increased vigour and strength. The isolation of testosterone was soon followed by the derivation of a series of synthetic anabolic steroids. This increased availability of anabolic steroids in the late 1960s introduced a set of drugs to sport that remain one of the most serious problems for anti-doping agencies to tackle.

Testosterone itself has two central properties: it is androgenic (it has the effect of developing masculine characteristics) and it is anabolic (it has a tissue-building effect). One motivation for the development of such a large number of synthetic steroids has been the attempt to separate the two effects and produce a steroid which is anabolic without also being androgenic. The search has so far proved fruitless and all steroids have both properties and are therefore properly referred to as androgenic-anabolic steroids (AAS).

The role of testosterone in developing male sexual characteristics occurs in two stages. During the early stages following conception testosterone is responsible for the development of primary male characteristics, while during puberty it affects the development of secondary sexual characteristics such as the development of pubic hair, enlarged testes and penis, a deeper voice and facial hair. Testosterone also has an effect on the behavioural characteristics associated with aggression. One of the main medical uses of androgenic anabolic steroids has been to treat problems associated with male development at puberty and thereby restore normal male secondary characteristics and normal male sexual behaviour. AAS have therefore been administered to accelerate the pubertal growth spurt, and they have also been used in the treatment of anaemia, renal failure and osteoporosis, as well as being used in the management of burn victims and to aid the recovery of patients from debilitating illnesses where there has been a loss of weight and strength.

The generally accepted view of the way in which steroids affect the body is that they increase protein synthesis. In brief, strength is proportionate to muscle bulk as measured by changes in the cross-sectional diameter of the muscle being evaluated. Muscle tissue is produced by the conversion of amino acids which are not produced by the body but are obtained by ingesting protein-rich food. Increasing the capacity of the body to create protein is only one of a number of theories which attempt to explain the real or imagined ergogenic effect of steroids. Other hypotheses include the suggestion that AAS enable a more effective utilisation of protein possibly through the increased production of insulin or growth hormone; that they enable more intense exercise to be undertaken which has the effect of stimulating muscle growth; or that the drugs are not inherently ergogenic but create a psychological state where harder and longer training is possible.

Steroids are almost certainly the most widely used drug in modern sport whether measured in terms of the number of countries where abuse has been discovered, the range of sports, and related activities in which steroids are deemed ergogenic, and the range of levels of competition where their use is apparent. Although steroids were first used by those sportsmen and women involved in sports that required strength or muscle mass, such as weightlifting, shot-put and discus, it was not long before the drug became common in the explosive events where athletes sought to increase their power. The perception that steroids provide an ergogenic advantage is widespread and deeply held and is best summed up in the report of the Dubin Inquiry:

> "The overwhelming evidence at this inquiry is that anabolic steroids enhance athletic performance. Witness after witness spoke of increased strength and size; of a greater ability to train intensely, to resist the pain of workouts, and to recuperate; of improved performances; and of new feelings of confidence, physical well-being, and enthusiasm. Coaches and physicians, who had the best opportunity to observe the athletes, were also unequivocal about the performance-enhancing effects which were evident primarily in events requiring weight and strength (including upper and lower body strength in sprinters)."[1]

Providing scientific corroboration for the widely held belief that steroids aid performance is difficult given that the quantities of steroids taken by athletes far exceeds that which would be ethically allowable in any controlled experiment. Use by athletes is often at levels ten to forty times the therapeutic level and may involve combining different steroids, referred to as "stacking", a practice in which the athlete uses a number of steroids with different pharmacological profiles usually in the hope of benefiting from assumed synergy between the drugs or else in the hope of avoiding the development of tolerance and therefore maintaining the impact of the drugs. In a recent survey it was found that 88% of steroid users practised "stacking".[2] Other regimes are referred to as "cycling" and "pyramiding". The former practice involves periods of intensive steroid use alternating with periods of abstinence and is designed to avoid some of the side effects of continuous steroid use. The latter practice is a variation on cycling and involves the gradual build up of drug use and an equally gradual decrease in use during each cycle.[3]

The evidence from scientific experiment indicates that steroids produce both physiological and psychological effects. There is a considerable volume of

1. Dubin Inquiry, "Commission of Inquiry into the Use of Drugs and Banned Practices Intended to Increase Athletic Performance", Ottawa, Canadian Government Publishing Centre, p. 103 (1990).
2. Evans, N.A. "Gym and Tonic, A Profile of 100 Male Steroid Users", *British Journal of Sports Medicine*, Vol. 31, pp. 54-58 (1997).
3. George, A. (1996) p. 182-3, op. cit.

experimental data concerning the physiological effects of steroids particularly regarding the effects on endurance, bulk and strength. While there seems to be a consensus that steroids have no impact on endurance,[1] there is a marked lack of consensus regarding the impact on bulk and strength. Numerous studies have concluded that steroids do increase strength,[2] with an equal number claiming no significant increase.[3] A survey of studies of the effects of steroids carried out between 1965 and 1977 concluded that there was "no substantial evidence" that steroid use in conjunction with progressive weight resistance training led to increased lean muscle bulk and greater strength.[4] On the contrary, there is a substantial body of evidence that will stand very close scrutiny to indicate that anabolic steroids will not contribute significantly to gains in lean muscle bulk or muscle strength in healthy young adult males.[5]

The conclusions of the survey suggested that the key factor undermining the ergogenic effect of steroids is the fact that the body compensates for any increase in steroid use by depressing the level of testosterone production. However, these conclusions are challenged by the argument that under particular circumstances steroids can be effective in increasing strength. Improvements will result if the athlete engages in intensive weight training before and during the course of steroids, consumes a high protein diet, and measurement of change is through single repetition weight techniques.[6] A similar conclusion was reached as a result of a 1984 survey which concluded that anabolic steroids can contribute to increases in lean mass and body weight if their use is supported by an adequate diet. It claimed that muscular strength could also be increased through the use of steroids if coupled with intensive training and proper diet. It also stated that steroids do not increase aerobic power[7] and suggested that the physiological effects of steroid use may, in part at least, be due to a placebo effect. In other words when athletes start taking steroids they expect to be able to train longer or lift heavier weights and consequently push themselves that much harder, attributing the improved performance

1. Fahey, T.D. & Brown, C.H., "The Effects of Anabolic Steroids on the Strength, Body Composition, and Endurance of College Males when Accompanied by a Weight Training Program", *Medicine and Science in Sports*, Vol. 5, pp. 272-276 (1973).
2. Stamford, B.A. & Moffatt, R., "Anabolic Steroid, Effectiveness as an Ergogenic Aid to Experienced Weight Trainers", *Journal Sports Med. Phys. Fitness*, Vol. 14, pp. 191-197, (1974); Ward, P. "The Effect of an Anabolic Steroid on Strength and Lean Body Mass", *Med. Sci. Sports*, Vol. 5, pp. 277-282 (1973).
3. Hervey, G.R., & Knibbs, A.V. et al, "Are Athletes Wrong About Anabolic Steroids?", *British Journal of Sports Medicine*, Vol. 9, pp. 74-77 (1975); Loughton, S.V. & Ruhline, R.O., "Human Strength and Endurance Responses to Anabolic Steroids and Training", *Journal Sports Med. Phys. Fitness*, Vol .17, pp. 285-296 (1977).
4. Ryan, A.J. "Anabolic Steroids are Fool's Gold", *Federation of American Society for Experimental Biology*, Vol. 40.12, pp. 2682-2688 (1981).
5. Ibid, p. 1684.
6. Haupt, H.A. & Rovere, G.D. "Anabolic Steroids, A Review of the Literature", *American Journal of Sports Medicine*, Vol. 12.6, pp. 469-484 (1984).
7. American College of Sports Medicine, "Stand on the Use of Anabolic-Androgenic Steroids in Sport", Indianapolis, American College of Sports Medicine (1984).

to the effects of the steroids rather than to their own determination and increased effort. Just such an effect was found in a study with experienced weightlifters who were told they were being given methandrostenolone, but were in fact receiving a placebo.[1] It is interesting to note that a very high proportion of illegally obtained steroids, which is a substantial proportion of the total used, is either fake or significantly adulterated. One survey found that 26% of a sample of thirty-four illegally obtained steroids tested contained no steroids, 53% were mislabelled and 85% contained the wrong dose.[2] These figures highlight the need for caution in accepting the conclusions of any study which is based on self-reporting by illegal steroid users.

The extended use of steroids has been associated with numerous side effects which range from the minor to the severe and which affect a variety of bodily systems. Because steroid use in men tends to depress the natural production of testosterone there are a number of side effects that affect sex organs and sexual behaviour. Testicular size tends to decrease as does the production of sperm.[3] The sex drive may also be affected, although the effect is variable, often producing an enhanced sex drive in the early stages of use but a diminished sex drive after sustained use.[4] A number of steroid users also take human chorionic gonadotrophin in an attempt to counteract testicular atrophy and/or diminished libido.[5] Additional problems may include the development of breast tissue.[6] Changes may also be experienced in the level of blood pressure and in the balance between high density and low density lipoprotein cholesterol: such changes have been identified as increasing the risk of cardiovascular disease.[7] While there is not sufficient evidence to draw a firm conclusion that changes in the cholesterol balance lead to increased cardiovascular risk, it is the case that in a review of sudden deaths among competitive athletes, three out of twenty-nine could be attributed to coronary atherosclerosis.[8]

---

1. Ariel, G & Saville, W., "Anabolic Steroids, the Physiological Effects of Placebos", *Medicine and Science in Sports*, Vol. 4, pp. 124-126 (1972).
2. Walters, M., Ayers, R. & Brown D., "Analysis of illegally distributed Steroid Products by Liquid Chromatography with Identity Confirmation by Mass Spectrometry or Infrared Spectrophotometry", *J Assoc. Off. Anal.Chem*, Vol. 73.6, pp. 904-926 (1990).
3. Jackson, H. & Jones, A.R., "The Effects of Steroids and their Antagonists on Spermatogenesis", *Adv. Steroid Biochem. Pharmacol.* Vol. 3 (1972).
4. Strauss, R.H., Wright, J.E, Finerman, G.A.M. & Catlin, D.H., "Side effects of Anabolic Steroids in Weight-trained Men", *Physician and Sports Medicine*, Vol. 11, pp. 87-101 (1983).
5. Ibid, p. 258.
6. Strauss, R.H., "Anabolic Steroids", in Strauss,R.H. (ed.), *Drugs and Performance in Sports*, Philadelphia, W.B. Saunders (1987).
7. See Rockhold, R.W., "Cardiovascular Toxicity of Anabolic Steroids", *Ann.Rev. Pharmac. Tox.*, Vol. 33, pp. 497-520 (1993) for a discussion of the evidence on the effect of steroids on blood pressure; Strauss, R.H., Wright, J.E, Finerman, G.A.M. & Catlin, D.H., "Anabolic Steroid Use and Health Status Among Weight Trained Male Athletes", *The Physician and Sports Medicine*, Vol. 13 (1985); McKillop, G. & Ballantyne, D. "Lipoprotein Analysis in Bodybuilders", *International Journal of Cardiology*, Vol. 17, pp. 281-281-286 (1987).
8. Ljungqvist, A. "Health Risks of Steroid Use", in Shipe, J.R. & Savory, J. (eds.), *Drugs in Competitive Athletics*, Oxford, Blackwell Scientific Publications (1991), p. 94.

For both men and women there have been reports of a risk of jaundice and liver damage, and also the danger that the self-administration of steroids may result in the transmission of diseases such as hepatitis B and Aids. A further concern is that steroid use may contribute to the likelihood of developing cancers of the liver.[1] Although a British weightlifter, Shaw, died in 1990 from liver tumours at the age of 25, the evidence is circumstantial rather than direct. There is also a series of side effects that affect women; a number of masculinising effects including a deepening of the voice, male pattern baldness, acne, growth of facial hair, changes or cessation of the menstrual function, decreased breast size and enlargement of the clitoris.[2]

Where use occurs among youths who have not yet fully matured the effects can be to accelerate the maturation process but to prevent the individual reaching his potential adult height.[3] However, the emergence of a scientific consensus on this particular side effect has been hampered by studies which suggest that some steroids can indeed by taken by boys to speed up growth without also accelerating skeletal maturation.[4]

In addition to the physiological side effects, there are also a number of psychological side effects including increased aggressiveness, sometimes referred to as "roid rages", and mood swings.[5] In one study, 22% of the sample of forty-one steroid users exhibited manic or depressive episodes at some time during their use of steroids.[6] Although these symptoms are serious they seem to disappear once the use of steroids has been discontinued.[7] But, contrary evidence suggests that prolonged use of steroids leads to addiction, especially among adolescent users.[8] It has also been suggested that depression has followed the cessation of steroid use.[9] Yet few of these conclusions can be seen as more than indicative as most are based on a very small sample or are individual case histories, often of the more dramatic cases. As a result, it is not possible to use the existing evidence as a basis for generalisation.

1. Vesselinovitch, S.D., Mihailovich, N. & Rao, K.V.N., "Potential Role of Synthetic Sex Steroids in Hepatocarcinogenesis", in Shipe, J.R. & Savory, J. (eds.), Drugs in Competitive Athletics, Oxford, Blackwell Scientific Publications (1991).
2. Ibid; Strauss, R. H., p. 483 (1984), op. cit.
3. Daniel, W.A. & Bennett, D.L. "The Use of Anabolic-androgenic Steroids in Childhood and Adolescence" in Kochakian, C.D. (ed.) Anabolic-androgenic Steroids, New York, Springer Verlag (1976); Lamb, D.R. "Anabolic Steroids in Athletics, How Well do they Work and How Dangerous are they?" American Journal of Sports Medicine, Vol. 12, pp. 31-38 (1984).
4. Millar, A.P., "Licit Steroid Use-Hope For the Future", British Journal of Sports Medicine, Vol. 28.2, pp. 79-83 (1994).
5. Ljungqvist, A. (1991), op. cit.
6. Pope, H.G. & Katz, D.L. "Affective and Psychotic Symptoms Associated with Anabolic Steroid Use", American Journal of Psychiatry, Vol. 145, pp. 487-490 (1988).
7. Bahrke, M.S., Yesalis, C.E. & Wright, J.E. "Psychological and Behavioral Effects of Endogenous Testosterone Levels and Anabolic Androgenic Steroids Among Males", Sports Medicine, Vol. 10, pp. 303-337 (1990).
8. Middleman, A.B. & DuRant, R.H. "Anabolic Steroid Use and Associated Health Risk Behaviours", Sports Medicine, Vol. 21.4, pp. 251-255 (1996).
9. Burkett, L.N. & Faldulto, M.T. "Steroid Use by Athletes in a Metropolitan Area", Physician and Sports Medicine, Vol. 12.8, pp. 69-74 (1984).

Although anabolic steroid dependency may be a problem, its prevalence and symptomology is difficult to establish reliably based upon the existing literature.[1] They also note that given the widespread use of steroids there seems to be a comparatively small number of cases of psychological conditions requiring treatment.

Despite the widespread assumption of a preoccupation among steroid users with their appearance and fitness, there is evidence of an association between steroid use and the abuse of other substances including cocaine and marijuana. Anabolic steroid use by young people has also been associated with other high-risk behaviour including driving while drunk, unprotected sex, and carrying a weapon.[2] In one of the most recent and comprehensive surveys of published data on the association between steroid use and a range of negative psychological effects, it was found that, apart from a small minority, most of the thirty-two studies confirmed the association.[3]

Testosterone

All that has been written about anabolic-androgenic steroids also applies to any discussion of testosterone. However, testosterone requires a brief separate discussion because of the recent increase in its abuse by athletes. Testosterone has been added to the IOC list of banned substances and practices only comparatively recently due to its increasing substitution for other anabolic steroids and because of the difficulties that doping agencies face in distinguishing exogenous from endogenous testosterone. The need to address the problem of testosterone abuse was highlighted at the 1980 Olympic Games where it was found that as many as two-thirds of all random urine samples contained abnormal levels of testosterone. As testosterone is produced within the body so too is a smaller amount of epitestosterone, its isomer. Because of differential rates of excretion the ratio of testosterone to epitestosterone is normally approximately 1:1. It is variation from this norm that provides the basis for identifying the presence of exogenous testosterone.

Testosterone is present in the bodies of both men and women. In pre-pubertal boys and women the level of daily production is less than 0.25 micrograms per day, while for men the level increases to between 2.5 micrograms and 11 micrograms per day with the surge in production taking place during puberty. In women testosterone is produced in the adrenal cortex and the ovaries: for men production is by the testes and also the adrenal cortex.

1. Bahrke, M.S., Yesalis, C.E. & Wright, J.E., "Psychological and Behavioral Effects of Endogenous Testosterone and Anabolic-Androgenic Steroids, An Update", *Sports Medicine*, Vol. 22.6, p. 384 (1996).
2. Middleman, A.B., Faulkner, A.H. & Woods, E.R. et al, "High Risk Behaviours Among High School Students in Massachusetts who use Anabolic Steroids", *Pediatrics*, Vol. 96, pp. 268-272 (1995)
3. Bahrke, M.S. et al (1996) op. cit.

Testosterone achieves its effects through a complex series of receptors distributed throughout the body.

The assumed value of testosterone to the athlete is similar to that of anabolic-androgenic steroids, namely having the physiological effect of promoting muscle growth and strength, and the psychological effect of enhancing aggression. As the use of exogenous testosterone is comparatively recent there are few studies which test its effectiveness in relation to sport. One of the few studies that have been carried out examined the effect of testosterone administered in weekly doses of 600 milligrams over a ten week period to males with experience of weight training.[1] The men were divided into four groups, the first received a placebo and took no exercise; the second group received doses of testosterone and took no exercise; the third was given a placebo coupled with resistance training; while the fourth group was given doses of testosterone coupled with resistance training. Both groups to whom testosterone was administered showed increases in muscle size and strength, but the greatest increase was evident among the group which was undertaking resistance training as well as receiving testosterone. There have also been some studies of the relationship between endogenous testosterone levels and mood and behaviour, one of which found a positive correlation between the level of aggressive behaviour in a sample of college students and levels of testosterone.[2] In one study it was found that men producing more testosterone are less likely to marry: once married, they are more likely to leave home because of troubled marital relations, extra-marital sex, hitting or throwing things at their spouses.[3] Although some studies question the link between aggression and testosterone levels, the balance of opinion is supportive of such a link and is one of the reasons for the choice of testosterone by drug abusers in sport. The psychological benefit in competition sought by abusers of testosterone is also one of the drug's main side effects, for although athletes hope to focus their enhanced levels of aggression on the competition it is impossible to prevent it spilling over into their non-sporting relationships.

Diuretics

Diuretics affect the rate at which urine is formed and directly affect the kidneys. Diuretics are used therapeutically to treat high blood pressure and excessive fluid retention. In sport these drugs have been used either to help achieve weight loss in weight-regulated sports such as wrestling and horse-racing, or to conceal the presence of other drugs by affecting the rate at which they are excreted in the urine. There is also evidence that body

---

1. Bhasin, S., Storer, T.W.. Berman, N. et al, "The Effects of Supra-physiologic doses of testosterone on muscle size and strength in normal men", *N. Eng. J. Med.*, Vol. 335, pp. 1-7 (1996).
2. Gladue, B. "Qualitative and Quantitative Sex Differences in Self-reported Aggressive Behavioural Characteristics" *Psychol. Rep.* Vol. 68, pp. 675-84 (1991).
3. Referred to in Bahrke, M.S. et al (1996), p. 372, op. cit.

builders are using diuretics in combination with steroids in order to counter-act the water-retention properties of the latter and, especially, to produce a sharper muscle definition by reducing the level of water retention. There are claims that diuretics can lead to an average weight loss of 4.1% within a twenty-four-hour period.[1] It is also claimed that the diuretic, acetazolamide, has the capacity to improve performance at high altitudes.[2]

The side effects of diuretic use are frequently difficult to isolate as the athlete is often either using other drugs which the diuretic is designed to help con-ceal or the athlete might be using other methods in addition to the diuretic to lose weight. The most obvious effect of diuretic use is dehydration which might not affect the athlete's performance in the early stages of competition but will usually affect performance in any sport which requires endurance. Because many diuretics also result in the excretion of potassium, there is a consequent risk of muscle cramps and general fatigue. In addition, "a stable level of potassium [...] is very important for muscular contractions, for the regularity and efficiency of the heartbeat".[3] The American College of Sports Medicine, in a paper on the effects on wrestlers of attempting to "make weight", identify a series of side effects including the following:

> "a reduction in muscle strength, (...) a decrease in work performance times, (...) lower plasma and blood volumes (...) a lower aerobic capacity (...) impairment of body temperature regulation (and) (...) a decrease in blood flow to the kidney and in the volume of fluid being filtered by the kidney."[4]

Peptide and glycoprotein and analogues

Human chorionic gonadatrophin

Human chorionic gonadatrophin (hCG) is produced in the placenta and in turn stimulates the production of the hormone progesterone during preg-nancy. When hCG is injected into males it has the effect of stimulating cells within the testis to produce testosterone and epitestosterone. The effect of hCG is rapid with reports that the production of plasma testosterone can be increased by 50% within two hours of injection.[5]

The attraction of hCG to drug abusers is that it possesses similar properties to steroids and, more importantly, is impossible to detect. The advantage of

1. Caldwell, J.E., Ahonen, E. & Nousiainen, U.; "Differential Effects of Sauna-, diuretic-, and exercise-induced hypohydration", *Journal of Applied Physiology*, Vol. 57 pp. 1018-1023 (1984).
2. Bradwell, A.R., Dykes, P.W., Coote, J.H. et al, "Effects of Acetazolamideon Exercise Perfor-mance and Muscle Mass at High Altitude", *Lancet*, Vol. 1.2, pp. 1001-05 (1986), quoted in Ver-roken, M. "Drug Use and Abuse in Sport" in Mottram, D.R. (1996), op. cit.
3. Comment from Dr Andrew Pipe giving evidence to the Dubin Inquiry p. 117, (1990). op. cit.
4. "Position Stand, Weight Loss in Wrestlers", American College of Sports Medicine, Indianapo-lis (1976).
5. Kicman, A.T., Brooks, R.V. & Cowan, D.A., "Human chorionic gonadotrophin and Sport", *British Journal of Sports Medicine*, Vol. 25 pp. 73-80 (1991).

hCG over both steroid abuse and testosterone abuse is that it stimulates the natural production of both testosterone and epitestosterone, thus keeping the ratio of testosterone to epitestosterone below the IOC threshold of 6:1.[1] The side effects of the drug are similar to those of steroids although one study has suggested that its use will prompt nausea and vomiting[2] and another noted that the incidence of the development of breast tissue may be greater due to the effect of the drug in stimulating the production of oestradiol.[3]

Adrenocorticotrophic hormone

Adrenocorticotrophic hormone (ACTH) is produced by the anterior pituitary and has the effect of stimulating the production of corticosteroids which have anti-inflammatory properties, and may also affect mood. However, the interest in ACTH among drug abusers in sport is focused on one of its derivatives, tetracosactrin, which stimulates a rise in blood cortisol and corticosterone concentration within two hours and is used in an attempt to reduce lethargy and produce "positive" effects on mood during training and competition.[4] It is claimed that the drug is used by cyclists to produce feelings of well-being or even euphoria.[5] However, the effects are not only short-lived but have the serious side effect of leading to wasting of the muscle if used over a long period. Because the use of synthetic ACTH suppresses the natural secretion of ACTH, there is a risk that a sharp reduction in drug use will result in an insufficiency of corticosteroids due to degeneration of the adrenal glands thus making the athlete more vulnerable to infection.

Human growth hormone

The increasing success of the doping agencies in detecting steroid abuse by athletes has encouraged some athletes to explore the potential benefits of human growth hormone (hGH). Human growth hormone is released from the pituitary gland and controls the natural growth of almost every body system. Its therapeutic use is to help growth hormone deficient children reach normal height. It has also been used successfully in helping growth in children who are not deficient in endogenous growth hormone.[6] Among the most important effects of hGH are to stimulate nitrogen retention (an important element in anabolic effects), to help break down fat and convert it to energy, and to stimulate the production of somatomedins, which are the

---

1. Ibid.
2. Goldman, B. (1992), op. cit.
3. George, A. "The Anabolic Steroids and Peptide Hormones", in Mottram, D.R. (1996), op. cit.
4. Ibid.
5. Donohoe, T. & Johnson, N (1986), p. 97, op. cit.
6. Van Vliet, G. et al "Growth Hormone Treatment for Short Stature", *New England Law Journal of Medicine*, Vol. 309, pp. 277-282 (1983).

molecules that facilitate growth. These findings have led to "the spurious thinking by some that providing human growth hormone to otherwise healthy athletes could result in considerable improvement in muscular strength (...) despite the fact that no scientific evidence exists that could document this effect in healthy individuals".[1]

Up until 1985 pituitary hGH was extracted from cadavers, but this was replaced by synthetic hGH when a number of children receiving treatment contracted Creutzfeldt-Jakob disease and subsequently died. The development of synthetic (genetically engineered) hGH coincided with an increase in its abuse by athletes who believed that, in addition to fulfilling the same role as anabolic steroids in producing muscle bulk and strength, it would also help to "prevent the breakdown of muscles after [A]AS use has been discontinued".[2] There was also a belief that hGH was able to strengthen tendons and ligaments thus reducing the likelihood of muscle damage during intensive training and competition.[3] Additional motives for using hGH included the assumption that it would enhance muscle growth but depress fat accumulation: it was also thought that some parents were supporting their children's use of hGH, if they were athletically able, in order to ensure that they reached the "approved or optimal" height for particular sports.[4] The paucity of experimental data makes confident generalisations about the effects of hGH impossible. Experiments on rats seem to indicate that hGH does enhance muscle bulk, especially in atrophied muscle. There is also some evidence that when hGH has been administered for therapeutic purposes to humans, muscle bulk has increased but not muscle strength. Wadler and Hainline support Puffer's conclusion by emphasising that no improved performance effect has ever been demonstrated from the use of this hormone.[5] This conclusion was further reinforced by a series of double-blind placebo controlled studies.[6] However, the combination of enthusiasm for the drug among athletes and a lack of evidence of any ergogenic value should come as no surprise as so much drug taking by athletes is based more on rumour and desperation than evidence.

---

1. Puffer, J.C. p. 82 (1986), op. cit.; see also Cowart, V.S., "Human Growth Hormone, The Latest Ergogenic Aid?", *Physician and Sports Medicine*, Vol. 16, pp. 175-185 (1988).
2. Rickert, V.I., Pawlak-Morello, C, Sheppard, V. & Jay, M.S., "Human Growth Hormone, A New Substance of Abuse Among Adolescents?", *Clinical Pediatrics*, Vol. 31, pp. 724 (1992).
3. Ibid.
4. Wadler, G.I. & Hainline, B. (1989), op. cit.
5. Ibid, p. 73. Very small reductions in fat and equally small increases in lean tissue have been suggested in a study by Crist, D.M., Peake, G.T., Egan, P.A., & Waters, D.L., "Body Composition Response to Exogenous GH During Training in Highly Conditioned Adults", *J App. Physiol.*, Vol. 65, p. 579-84 (1988).
6. Deyssig, R., Frisch, H., Blum, W.F. et al , "Effects of Growth Hormone Treatment on Hormonal Parameters, Body Composition and Strength in Athletes, *Acta Endocrinol.*, No. 128, pp. 313-8, (1993) ;Tarasheki, K.E., Campbell, J.A., Smith, K., Rennie, M.J., Holloway, J.O. & Bier, D.M., "Effect of Growth Hormone and Resistance exercise on Muscle Growth in Young Men", *Am. J. Physiol. Endocrinol. Metab.*, Vol. 262, E261-7 (1992).

Just as there is little research into the ergogenic effects of hGH, whether natural or synthetic, there is also little research evidence regarding the possible side effects of the abuse of the synthetic hGH which is currently available. The evidence that exists is based on the side effects of naturally occurring over-secretion of growth hormone and includes the over-growth of bones (particularly of the jaw, forehead and fingers) and soft tissue, and coronary artery disease. In addition, as hGH must be injected there is the risk of infections, such as Aids and hepatitis B, from dirty needles.

Doping methods

Blood doping: transfusion and rEPO

Blood doping by transfusion involves the removal of blood (approximately one litre) from the athlete whereupon the red blood cells are separated from the plasma and preserved. Following the removal of the blood the athlete's red blood cell count will return to normal. Once this has been achieved (four to six weeks later) the preserved red blood cells are reintroduced into the athlete. Because the amount of oxygen that an athlete can make available to muscle tissue is limited by the number of red blood cells, the overall effect of blood doping by transfusion is to increase the red blood cell count and thereby increase the amount of oxygen available to the muscles. The same effect can also be achieved by the introduction of blood from another person with a compatible blood type. The use of another's blood is by far the most common form of blood doping by transfusion as the cost of an athlete using his or her own blood is higher due to the more sophisticated laboratory requirements.

The transfusion of half a litre of blood can provide the athlete with about an additional half litre of oxygen to the muscle per minute.[1] In addition, there is evidence that not only does blood doping by transfusion increase the flow of oxygen to the muscle but it also has the effect of increasing the volume of oxygen actually used during intense exercise.[2] The practice of blood doping by transfusion is attractive because the ergogenic effects are evident almost immediately and are of especial value in endurance events such as cycling and running. The effect of blood doping by transfusion is similar to that achieved naturally through high altitude training.

Initially there was some scepticism about the ergogenic value of blood doping by transfusion. The explanation for the failure of early experiments to produce quantifiable gains was due to the weaknesses in technique which, once sufficiently refined, was able to demonstrate verifiable ergogenic advantage. According to evidence given to the Dubin Inquiry, blood doping by transfusion has the potential to increase the maximal capacity to use

---

1. Wadler, G.I. & Hainline, B. (1989), op. cit.
2. Robertson, R.J. et al, "Hemoglobin Concentration and Aerobic Work Capacity in Women Following Induced Erythrocythemia", *Journal of Applied Physiology*, Vol. 57 (1984).

oxygen by 5%.[1] Other studies have confirmed the benefits of blood doping by transfusion with one reporting that athletes participating in a 10-kilometre run were able to sustain greater speed during the later stages of races and could therefore improve their times by over one minute.[2] However, the benefit from blood doping by transfusion is greater for those athletes that have a high level of initial fitness.

There are a number of potential side effects associated with blood doping by transfusion that arise from the use of blood which is not the athlete's own, including infections such as Aids, and reactions to incompatible blood. In addition, the increase in the volume of blood in the body may cause a dangerous increase in blood pressure.

Training at altitude can have a similar effect to blood doping by transfusion. The effect of altitude training is to prompt an increase in the natural synthesis of erythropoietin due to the reduction of oxygen at greater altitudes and the body's consequent need to adjust in order to maintain its effectiveness. The recognition of the process of acclimatisation has encouraged experimentation with synthetic erythropoietin (rEPO). Synthetic erythropoietin's availability dates from 1984 when the American pharmaceutical company Amgen was granted a patent for its production. Its main medical use is to help patients suffering from a range of serious illnesses including renal disease, some cancers and anaemia. rEPO was added to the IOC list of banned substances in 1990 even though a secure method for its detection was not then available. As regards the effects of the drug on sportsmen and women, the administration of rEPO has a pronounced effect on the aerobic performance of endurance athletes, once time is allowed for the over-stimulation of the bone marrow to have its effect.[3]

Although the broad effect of the administration of rEPO is the same as that found for blood doping by transfusion, it is far more difficult to predict the consequences of the use of the drug. In particular, prediction of the scale of increase in the production of red blood cells is much less accurate. As a result there is a heightened risk of dangerously elevated levels of blood pressure and blood viscosity with the increased risk of thrombosis and stroke.[4]

---

1. Dubin Inquiry (1990), p. 121, op. cit.; Gledhill, N., "Blood doping and Related Issues, A Brief Review", *Med. Sci. Sports Exerc.* Vol. 14.3 (1983). See also Buick et al who demonstrated that the practice can lead to significant improvements in maximal oxygen consumption and total exercise time among elite runners. Buick, F.J., Gledhill, N. & Froese, A.B. et al, "Effect of Induced Erythrocythemia on Aerobic Work Capacity", *Journal of Applied Physiology*, Vol. 48, pp. 636-642 (1980).
2. Brien, T. & Simon, T.L. ,"The Effects of Red Blood Cell Infusion on 10km Race Time", Journal of the American Medical Association, Vol. 257, pp. 2761-5 (1987).
3. Armstrong, D.J. & Reilly, T., "Blood boosting and Sport", in Mottram, D.R. (1996), op. cit.; for an estimate of the value of rEPO see also Eachbach, J.W. et al ,"Correction of the Anemia of End-stage Renal Disease with Recombinant Human Erythropoietin. Results of a Combined Phase I and II Clinical Trial", *New England Journal of Medicine*, Vol. 316 (1987).
4. Ibid.

Pharmacological, chemical and physical manipulation

The ingenuity and effort that some athletes and their coaches put into attempts to obtain an unfair advantage through the use of drugs is matched only by their equal investment in seeking ways to disguise the fact that doping has taken place. The IOC Medical Commission, therefore, in 1985 introduced regulations to cover attempts to deceive testing authorities. The most common examples of deception are urine substitution and the inhibition of renal excretion.

There are a number of ways in which urine manipulation and substitution can take place. Athletes may, for example, store sufficient urine taken at a time when they were not using drugs and use a catheter to reintroduce it into their bladder prior to a drug test. Perhaps the best known example of urine manipulation concerned three German athletes, Grit Breuer, Katrin Krabbe and Silke Müller, who were tested while in South Africa for training. The urine samples they provided were so similar that it was alleged that they had come from the same person, possibly as a result of catheterisation.

Attempts to inhibit renal excretion often involve the use of the drug probenecid, normally used for the treatment of gout as a means of delaying the excretion of antibiotics and thereby prolonging their therapeutic effectiveness. The effect of probenecid and other similar drugs (such as carinamide) is to prevent the excretion of certain other drugs, particularly steroids, so that an ostensibly clean urine sample can be given.

Classes of drugs subject to certain restrictions

Alcohol

Alcohol is probably the most common and socially acceptable drug. Its use is a cause for concern in some sports such as motor racing, downhill skiing and ski jumping not because of any claimed advantage that it confers but because of the threat to the athlete's safety or the safety of other participants. There is also an awareness in higher risk sports that the public image of the sport would be tarnished by accidents and particularly alcohol-related accidents. More widely, the link between sport and alcohol is a cause of concern due to its association with poor standards of crowd behaviour or with patterns of social behaviour that have developed in some sports. In general, alcohol is of value in only a limited number of sports. In the 1970s, there were some claims that some alcoholic products, beers in particular, were good sources of carbohydrates and were also useful ways of replenishing lost body fluid caused by training for competition. But beer is an inefficient source of carbohydrate and also, due to alcohol's diuretic effect, an equally inefficient source of replacement fluid.[1]

---

1. O' Brien, C.P., "Alcohol and Sport", Sports Medicine, Vol. 15.2, pp. 71-77 (1993).

It is common knowledge that the impact of alcohol on the body varies dramatically according to the amount consumed. Because even moderate amounts impair most sports-related functions, research into the potential value of alcohol consumption in sport has focused on the effects of relatively small amounts. Alcohol affects the body primarily through the central nervous system and reduces tension felt by athletes in stressful situations. Alcohol can produce feelings of mild euphoria, but also depression (normally as a result of the consumption of moderate to large amounts). The effect of alcohol use in sport is limited. Although one study demonstrated that moderate amounts of alcohol could lead to an increase in strength, there is considerable scepticism at this finding which has proved difficult to replicate.[1] There is little recent evidence that alcohol, even in moderate to low amounts, has any value in improving strength or endurance.

It is generally considered that the main value of alcohol is in those sports that require a steady aim, such as shooting, snooker, darts and archery.[2] In a detailed study of the effect of alcohol on accuracy in archery, arm steadiness, isometric strength, muscular endurance and reaction time was measured among nine archers when sober, when receiving a placebo and when receiving two different doses of alcohol. The results showed no effect on either isometric strength or muscular endurance, and a worsening of both reaction time and arm steadiness. Although the authors accepted that the results might have been different if the study had been conducted under competition conditions, the results provide an important challenge to the assumed benefits of low to moderate level alcohol use.[3] The study adds weight to the summary of available research provided which concludes that alcohol impairs all the following skills: balance and steadiness, reaction time, fine and complex motor co-ordination, visual tracking and information processing.[4]

Marijuana

Marijuana is similar to alcohol in that the main concern of anti-doping authorities is its association with sport, and especially the consequences for the image of sport of its recreational use by athletes, rather than its ergogenic value in sport. Marijuana is also similar to alcohol insofar as it is a depressant that operates through the central nervous system.

If alcohol's value as an ergogenic drug is, at best, limited, it is difficult to identify any significant ergogenic properties for marijuana. The main physiological effects of the drug are to increase blood pressure and the resting heart

---

1. Ikai, M. & Steinhaus, A.H., "Some Factors Modifying the Expression of Human Strength", *Journal of Applied Physiology*, Vol. 16 (1961).
2. Koller, W.C. & Biary, N. "Effect of Alcohol on Tremors, Comparison with Propanolol", *Neurology*, Vol. 34, pp. 221-222 (1984).
3. Reilly, T. & Halliday, F., "Influence of Alcohol Ingestion on Tasks Related to Archery", *J. Hum. Ergol.*, Vol. 14, pp. 252-8 (1985).
4. Wadler, G.I & Hainline, B., p. 128 (1989), op. cit.

rate without any beneficial effect on sports-related capacities, such as strength, fine-motor co-ordination, alertness or endurance.[1] Some athletes value marijuana for its capacity to reduce tension prior to and during competition.[2]

At low doses it causes sedation and euphoria while at high doses there is a risk of hallucinations and psychosis. Chronic use of the drug has been associated with a decline in motivation and also decreased testosterone levels.[3]

Corticosteroids

Corticosteroids are quite distinct from anabolic steroids. Synthetic corticosteroids are powerful anti-inflammatory drugs which mimic the effects of the corticosteroids produced naturally by the adrenal gland at times of stress. The primary medical use of corticosteroids is as analgesics (particularly in treatment of rheumatoid arthritis) and for the treatment of asthma.

The main use of corticosteroids in sport is to treat localised injury and pain. Used as a short-term treatment for injury, the corticosteroids can be very effective. However, where they are used over the longer term there are a number of side effects, such as osteoporosis and weakening of muscles.[4]

Beta-blockers

Beta-blockers are drugs which are designed to affect the body's beta adrenergic receptors, of which there are two types. Beta-1 receptors mediate cardiac effects while beta-2 receptors mediate bronchodilatation and the dilation of the blood vessels. There are also two types of beta-blocker, those which are non-selective and which therefore affect beta-1 and beta-2 receptors, and selective beta-blockers which affect beta-1 receptors. Beta-blockers are used in the treatment of a variety of conditions including angina, cardiac arrhythmias, migraine, tremor and a variety of anxiety-related symptoms. The drugs function by decreasing the heart rate, the degree of contraction of blood vessels around the heart, and systemic arterial blood pressure.

The main use of beta-blockers in sport is in those events where steadiness of the hand or arm is required such as shooting, golf, archery and snooker. The selective beta-blocker, metoprolol, has been shown to improve accuracy in shooting, with the benefit being greatest among the better shots,[5] and to have improved the shooting scores in twenty-two out of thrity-three

1. Steadward, R.D & Singh, M., "The Effects of Smoking Marijuana on Physical Performance", *Medicine and Science in Sport*, Vol. 7, pp. 309-311 (1975).
2. Wagner, J.C., "Abuse of Drugs used to Enhance Athletic Performance", *American Journal of Hospital Pharmacy*, Vol. 8, pp. 832-834 (1989).
3. Schwenk, T.L., p. 37 (1997), op. cit.
4. Elliot, P. "Drug Treatment of Inflammation in Sports Injuries", in Mottram, D.R. (1996), op. cit.
5. Schwenk, T.L., p. 40 (1997), op. cit.

participants.[1] Beta-blockers appear to be of value in only a narrow range of sports, as the drugs also have the effect of adversely affecting both aerobic and anaerobic endurance, partly as a result of the reduction in the maximum oxygen uptake. For example, the time taken to run 5000 metres was increased by 33% following the use of metoprolol.[2] Although endurance is affected, other capacities including muscle strength and power remain unaffected.[3] However, some athletes have tried to counter this by taking beta-blockers that had a shorter life and would be metabolised before the endurance element or event commenced. In addition, there is a risk that the capacity of the drug to result in peripheral constriction of the blood vessels may cause poor blood supply to the fingers which, particularly in winter, can cause considerable pain.

The side effects of beta-blockers can be serious, especially in those with existing cardiac problems for whom beta-blockers may cause heart failure. Other side effects include breathing problems and impotence. Some of the non-selective beta-blockers, especially those that are able to relieve anxiety most rapidly also tend to cause insomnia, nightmares and depression. There is also concern at the possible withdrawal symptoms which can manifest as anxiety, palpitations, angina, excessive sweating and headaches.[4]

Conclusion

This brief review of the drugs and practices banned or restricted by the IOC and other major sports organisations indicates not only the variety of substances and activities that the anti-doping authorities seek to control but also the scale of the problem they face. The development of policy and testing arrangements would be much more straightforward if the problem to be tackled was static, if the number of drugs and the ways in which they were administered remained constant. Unfortunately, as with many other social problems, doping in sport is dynamic and complex. Its dynamism arises from the steady development of new drugs, the constant exploration of the wealth of existing drugs for those with as yet undiscovered ergogenic properties, and the constant refinement of existing preparations. The complexity of the problem arises from issues of definition, and co-ordination between agencies, as much as from problems of detection and prosecution.

Table 3.1 provides an overview of the problem of doping in sport and highlights a number of issues. The second column makes clear the extent to which the drugs of abuse are not those that are easily available. Apart from

---

1. Kaiser, P. "Physical Performance and Muscle Metabolism During beta-adrenergic Blockade in Man", *Acta Physiologica Scandinavica*, Vol. 536 (Supplement), pp. 1-53 (1984).
2. Armstrong, D.J., "Sympathomimetic Amines and their Antagonists" in Mottram, D.R. (1996), op. cit.
3. Tesch, P.A. "Exercise Performance and Beta-blockade", *Sports Medicine*, Vol. 2, pp. 389-412 (1985).
4. Goldman (1992), p. 179, op. cit.

Table 3.1: Drugs in sport: a summary of their uses and side effects

Drug	Common legal classification	Main medical uses	Extent of use in sport	Strength of evidence of ergogenic value	Side effects
Amphetamine	controlled	relief of mild depression, treatment of narcolepsy, and control of appetite	considerable	strong	extensive and moderately serious
Cocaine	controlled	very slight; some use as a topical anaesthetic	moderate	negligible	extensive and extremely serious
Ephedrine	controlled, except when used in OTC preparations	element in many OTC cold and cough remedies; also used in some asthma and hay fever preparations	considerable	strong	moderate
Caffeine	legal	very slight; some use in the treatment of migraine; also present in some OTC analgesic preparations	slight to moderate	debatable, though the balance of opinion suggests some value in endurance sports	serious
Morphine	controlled	relief of severe pain; some use in the treatment of diarrhoea	slight	strong	extensive and extremely serious
Anabolic-androgenic steroids	controlled	treatment of anaemia, growth problems, renal failure	considerable	moderate to strong	extensive and moderately serious
Diuretics	controlled	treatment of high blood pressure and excessive fluid retention	slight	no ergogenic value, but evidence of value as a "weight reducing" agent	varied and moderately severe
hCG	controlled	testosterone deficiency	considerable	strong	moderate to severe
hGH	controlled	treatment of human growth deficiency, osteoporosis and potentially obesity	slight to moderate	weak	severe
ACTH	controlled	anti-inflammatory treatment	largely unknown, but probably slight	weak	severe
Blood doping	legal	none	considerable	strong	moderate to severe
Alcohol	legal	none	slight during competition	weak	only significant with heavy and/or long term use
Marijuana	controlled	negligible	considerable	almost none, use is primarily recreational	only significant with heavy and/or long term use
Beta-blockers	controlled	treatment of angina, migraine and tremor	slight to moderate	moderate to strong	in general only severe if pre-existing cardiac problem

alcohol and caffeine the other common drugs of abuse are, in most countries, controlled by the state. Some drugs, such as human growth hormone, are controlled very tightly by both the state and the producers: others, such as cocaine and heroin, are at the centre of multimillion-dollar police campaigns to reduce supply, with the imposition of substantial punishments for those caught possessing, and especially, supplying the drugs. The picture is more varied for the ingredients of common medical drugs such as steroids and beta-blockers, but even these are usually subject to some restrictions. While it is clear that some drugs can be purchased openly, many require a high degree of collusion between producers, chemists, doctors and coaches in order for them to be available to the athlete.

The last three columns describe the impact of research evidence on the extent of use. In general, and as one would expect, there is a reasonably close relationship between the extent of use and the strength of scientific evidence of ergogenic value. However, there is a far looser relationship between the extent of use and the seriousness of the possible side effects confirming the frequently made point that athletes have a limited regard for their own long term health and are willing to take considerable risks to achieve success. The problems remain of devising and implementing an anti-doping policy which has to be sensitive to a wide range of factors including the differing legal status of the drugs on the IOC list. The active collusion of a broad range of professionals is counterbalanced with the paradoxical willingness of athletes who depend on good health for sporting success to risk their medium to long-term wellbeing.

Chapter 4

Beyond sport: doping and anti-doping policy

The practice of sport and the men and women involved in it are as much a part of society as those involved in any other social pastime or occupation. This is not to suggest that the expectation that sportsmen and women should aspire to higher moral standards is misplaced, but rather to recognise that sport is not insulated from broader social values. However, simply to state the truism that there is a relationship between the culture of drug use in sport and that found in society does little to explain the nature of that interrelationship. Figure 4.1 attempts to illustrate the character of that relationship and provides a context for the discussion of policy issues.

Figure 4.1: A variety of contexts for drug use in sport

Sport: competitive; formal; elite-led; career oriented; commercial	Many Olympic sports particularly in track and field	Major international sports (Olympic Games a less central focus): e.g. soccer, cricket, golf, squash	Non-Olympic commercial sports: motor racing, American football, snooker, body building	Non-Olympic and substantially non-commercial sports: e.g. lacrosse, fishing and hunting	Competitive, commercial, non-sports: e.g. professional wrestling, "Gladiators", and strength competitions	Loosely organised, non-competitive sports-related activities: e.g. keep-fit, jogging clubs, aerobics, calisthenics	Unorganised, individual, non-sports-oriented activities: e.g. vanity body building	Sport: non-competitive; informal; mass; non-career oriented; non-commercial

Dividing sport from non-sport or sport from society is not easy. There have been many attempts to define sport and particularly to distinguish it from spectacle, entertainment, pastime and games with most attempts highlighting the extent to which sport as an activity is blurred at the boundary. It is necessary to explore the boundary of anti-doping policy for sport and the relationship between this policy and that for drug abuse in wider society. How are policies adopted to reduce the social and recreational use of drugs? How can we identify the lessons that might be learnt by those responsible for the implementation of anti-doping policy in sport?

Figure 4.1 presents an ideal continuum of sporting contexts for drug use which, for heuristic purposes, presents a view of sport which at one extreme emphasises a competitive, formal and elite-centred activity, but also one which provides the elite at least with an income-earning career within an increasingly commercial context. At the other extreme are those drug-using activities whose association with sport is at best tangential and which are non-competitive, informal, mass, non-career oriented, and often take place in a non-commercial context. Two further characteristics that overlay the continuum are the organisational context within which the activity takes place. This ranges from formal domestic sports organisations and international federations towards the left-hand side of the continuum, moving through progressively looser and less formal bodies such as professional associations, short-term event-organising bodies to informal and local organisations, and finally to personal initiative at the other extreme. The second characteristic concerns the range of motives that lead to drug use. Although it is acknowledged that motives for involvement in different types of sport will be multiple and shifting for those participating in the more formal and commercial sports, primary motives for drug use are likely to include the desire to improve the quality of performance and the chances of victory linked to a concern to retain employment and ensure participation. For those involved in informal and individualised "sporting" activities, significant motives are likely to include the enhancement of self-esteem or social success.

Current anti-doping policy in sport is derived from two sources, from among a range of sports organisations and from governments. Not surprisingly, the focus of sports organisation has been on formal competitive sport typified by participation in the Olympic Games or in one of the major international team sports. The IOC and the major international federations affiliated to GAISF (the General Association of International Sports Federations) have been the lead bodies in policy development supported by a range of governments and governmental organisations, including the Council of Europe. Understandably the sports organisations have focused narrowly on the problem of doping within their own particular sports or within the major multisport competitions, such as the Olympics, in which their athletes take part. Less attention has been paid to the broad range of sports on the fringe of Olympic and major team sports such as competitive body building, power-lifting, strongman/ woman competitions. Less attention still has been paid to the informal fringe sports-like activities such as keep-fit, aerobics and vanity body building where the motive is more likely to be social or psychological (to enhance self-esteem or sexual attraction). The use of "sports" drugs for social and psychological motives has as much in common with the broader issue of the recreational use of drugs as it has with doping in sport and it is at this end of the spectrum of drug use that governments have their primary interest, focus their resources and have the greatest accumulation of experience. Consequently, where the focus of government concern is broad, that of the sports federations and the IOC is narrow; where government experience is with the control of illegal drugs, that of the sports organisations is with legal, controlled and illegal drugs; and where governments deploy a variety of resources including the law and extensive police, welfare and medical services, the sports organisations rely on regulation and limited educational, medical and scientific services.

Although one can appreciate the narrowness of focus of the IOC and the international federations, the boundary between what might be referred to as mainstream sport (Olympic and major team sport) and fringe sport (such as body building, and exhibition/ novelty sports events) is frequently indistinct with athletes often crossing the boundary more than once in their lives. Attitudes and policy towards drug use are not neatly compartmentalised, and it is therefore important to understand the extent and character of drug use on the fringes of mainstream sport and beyond. Just as athletes will move between sporting activities, they also move, even when concentrating on elite competition, between the focused activities of intense training and competition and the social milieu that elite and frequently wealthy athletes inhabit. Both these patterns of movement, represented in Figure 4.2, bring athletes into contact with a variety of work and social situations which have different drug cultures which are not discrete but overlap and influence each other, each varying in terms of the preferred drugs, range of drugs used, sophistication and intensity of use. Consequently, the policy response of sports authorities and governments must, on the one hand, recognise the particular characteristics and environment of a series of drug-abusing communities while also, on the other hand, acknowledging the extent to which they overlap and drug abusers may move from one community to another.

Figure 4.2 : Drug-abusing communities

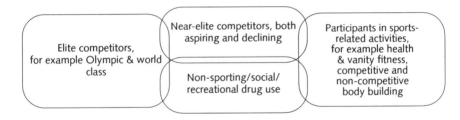

A further complication is the extent to which drug-dependent cultures have become established in the richer industrial countries. While the particular drug sub-cultures associated with participation in elite sport or body building may be seen as embedded in a broader sub-culture of illegal drug use, that sub-culture is itself embedded in a wider culture which has become, over the last thirty years or so, increasingly drug tolerant, dependent and obsessed. It is often argued that we are an increasingly drug-obsessed society where pharmaceutical solutions are sought not simply for medical complaints, but also for situations and activities that are a normal part of social life. Those who want to lose weight look to drugs rather than to dietary control and increased exercise; those seeking to avoid jet-lag take drugs; and those women who want to control their fertility take drugs. How can we expect potential drug abusers in sport to reconcile the contradictory messages that drugs should be shunned while also telling them that drugs are increasingly the primary and preferred solution to a range of medical and social conditions? Dr Andrew Pipe suggests that "In years gone by, men used to mistake magic for medicine, now men mistake medicine for magic".[1]

The change in social attitudes to medicine and the products of pharmaceutical companies is simply the outcome of a process which has been termed "the medicalisation of life" which has progressively blurred the distinction between health and illness.[2] Over recent years there has been a steady broadening of the range of human conditions that have been defined as medical problems such as ageing, pregnancy, alcoholism and, interestingly, drug addiction. Both ageing and pregnancy are examples of normal processes that have become problems that require medical expertise and treatment, while until very recently alcoholism and drug addiction were regarded as eccentricities that required care rather than illnesses that required cure. An increasing proportion of life events and conditions have become diagnosable, making the phrases that we use to describe them, such as healthy pregnancy, normal puberty, and growing old gracefully appear oxymorons. Waddington argues that this process of medicalisation has embraced sport and quotes the author of one of the first medical texts to focus on sports medicine as suggesting that "Just as extreme youth and senility produce peculiar medical problems, so too does extreme physical fitness".[3] Once it is accepted that extreme physical fitness makes an athlete by definition a patient then there is already in existence a culture, professionally supported and promoted, that encourages the treatment of healthy athletes with drugs. Even if the "drugs" are simply those which are legally available (in terms defined by both the state and the IOC), such as vitamins and food supplements, the athlete is already developing the expectations and patterns of behaviour that might initially parallel illegal drug use, but which are to most athletes part of a common culture. Robert Voy, former chief medical officer for the US Olympic Committee, illustrates this point very clearly when he recorded the daily intake of legal drugs that a national track star was taking: vitamin E, 160mg; B-complex capsules, four times per day; vitamin C, 2000 mg; vitamin B6, 150 mg; calcium tablets, four times per day; magnesium tablets, twice a day; zinc tablets, three times a day; royal jelly capsules; garlic tablets; cayenne tablets; eight aminos; Gamma-Oryzanol; Mega Vit Pack; supercharge herbs; Dibencozide; glandular tissue complex; natural steroid complex; Inosine; Orchic testicle extract; Pyridium; Ampicillin; and hair rejuvenation formula with Biotin.[4]

1. Goldman, B. & Klatz, R., *Death in the Locker Room II*, Chicago, Elite Sports Medicine Publications (1992), p. 18.
2. This section draws on an excellent article by Ivan Waddington "The Development of Sports Medicine", *Sociology of Sport Journal*, Vol. 13, pp. 176-196 (1996).
3. Ibid., p. 179. The quote is from Williams, J.G.P., *"Sports Medicine"*, London, Edward Arnold (1962).
4. Voy, R., "Drugs, Sport and Politics, The Inside Story about Drug Abuse in Sport and its Political Cover-up", Champaign, Ill., Leisure Press (1991), p. 99.

A further source of ambiguity arises from the intimate involvement of the medical and scientific professions in the development, and refinement in the use, of drugs. Mention has already been made of the central role of Dr Zeigler in identifying and disseminating information on the use of steroids among weightlifters, and of the Ciba Pharmaceutical Company in producing steroids. However, by far the clearest example of medical and scientific involvement in doping concerns the former German Democratic Republic (GDR). Writing in a confidential report in 1977, the Deputy Director of the Sports Medical Service[1], Manfred Höppner commented that "At present anabolic steroids are applied in all Olympic sporting events, with the exception of sailing and gymnastics (female)."[2] The total number of elite athletes treated each year exceeded 2000, a number which was augmented by the large number of second-rank athletes and juniors who were also treated.

Clearly such an extensive doping programme could not have been carried out without the close involvement of the state and the medical and scientific communities. The government of the GDR successfully shrouded the experimentation and administration of steroids under the cloak of state security and thereby maintained a remarkable level of secrecy. Scientists and doctors at the three research centres in Saxony, Leipzig and Kreischa worked closely with scientists at the state-owned pharmaceutical company, VEB Jenapharm, which developed the most widely used androgenic-anabolic steroid Oral-Turinabol in the mid 1960s. In the early 1980s it was also VEB Jenapharm which developed and produced preparations of epitestosterone propionate, a biologically inactive compound that had no commercial value but was prepared exclusively for the government doping system and whose function was to bring the testosterone – epitestosterone ratio back to the norm.[3] Such was the scale of involvement of doctors and scientists in the East German doping programme that it was observed that the "role that scientists and physicians have played in this clandestine system is particularly sad, not only because these professionals actively contributed to worldwide cheating, but also because they violated scientific and medical ethics".[4]

In addition to those doctors and scientists who were involved directly in doping programmes, there are also those medical professionals who appear, at best, ambivalent about the use of drugs in sport: there "are no overriding ethical reasons that force one to conclude that drug taking by an individual

---

1. Sportmedizinscher Dienst (SMD).
2. Quoted in Franke, W.W. & Berendonk, B., "Hormonal doping and androgenization of athletes, a secret program of the German Democratic Republic government", *Clinical Chemistry*, Vol. 43.7, pp. 1262-1279 (1997). Franke & Berendonke note that the exclusion of female gymnastics from the anabolic steroid programme was reversed in 1979 when female gymnasts were systematically treated with mestanlone.
3. Franke, W.W. & Berendonk, B., op. cit., p. 1272.
4. Ibid., p. 1263.

sportsman is necessarily unethical, or that the governing bodies of sport must have rules to prevent and punish drug taking".[1]

The evolution of the medical profession and the steady expansion of its sphere of competence in society, coupled with the increasing pressures from governments and commerce on athletes to succeed, has consequently led to a deepening relationship between the athlete and the doctor (and other sports scientists) and, for most athletes, a growing dependence. Thus the complaint voiced by an American runner who finished second that "I need a better doctor" may well represent a typical attitude among elite athletes.[2]

Body building and drug use

One activity which can be found in a variety of forms at various points across the continuum in Figure 4.1 is body building. At one extreme body building can be seen as closely linked to the Olympic sport of weightlifting, if not in terms of goals and skills then certainly in terms of similarity of many training techniques, equipment and facilities. Body building has many of the attributes of mainstream sport and, in many countries, has an elaborate, well-organised and tightly regulated competition circuit. At the less structured end of the continuum, body building shades into a more generalised weight-training activity directed at the development and maintenance of general fitness. Less structured still is the participation in body building activities for motives not associated with sport or even fitness and health, but more with vanity and narcissism, a pre-occupation with appearance and peer group esteem.

Within mainstream sport, weightlifting has suffered a number of drug-related scandals, probably best illustrated by the evidence given during the Dubin Inquiry in Canada. It should, therefore, come as no surprise that drug abuse is substantial within competitive, fitness and vanity body building. In a survey of 138 male body builders, 38% had used anabolic steroids.[3] Similar results have been found in surveys of steroid use among body builders in Wales, where 50% reported steroid use and in Kansas and Missouri where the total was 54%.[4] In a review of doping amongst body builders in the Flanders region of Belgium, reference was made to 'the widespread doping plague in body builders'.[1] Doping control became the responsibility of the Flemish Min-

---

1. Nicholson, R.H. "Drugs in Sport", *National Rifle Association Journal*, Vol. LXVI.3 (1987).
2. Quoted in Mangi, R.J. & Jokl, P. "Drugs and Sport", *Conn. Med.* Vol. 45, pp. 637-641 (1981).
3. Lindstrom, M., Nilsson, A., Katzman, P. et al, "Use of Anabolic Androgenic Steroids Among Body Builders - Frequency and Attitudes", *J. Intern. Med.*, Vol. 227, pp. 407-11 (1990).
4. Perry, H.M., Wright, D. & Littlepage, B.N.C., "Dying to be Big, A Review of Anabolic Steroid Use", *British Journal of Sports Medicine*, Vol. 26, pp. 259-262 (1992); Tricker, R., O' Neill, M.R. & Cook, D., "The Incidence of Anabolic Steroid Use Among Competitive Body Builders", *Journal of Drug Education*, Vol. 19, pp. 313-325 (1989).

istry of Health in 1988 and in the subsequent five years it carried out 379 tests of which 159 (42%) were positive (see Table 4.1). The proportion of positives found among body builders is put into perspective when the figures are compared with the proportion of positives for all sports in the same region, which were 6.1%, 6.3% and 5.7% respectively for the years 1990, 1991 and 1992, when a total of approximately 1700 tests were conducted each year.

Table 4.1: Doping results among Flemish body builders, 1988-93

Date	Number of tests	Number of positives	% positives
1988	32	7	22
1989	16	2	13
1990	42	29	69
1991	99	35	35
1992	82	41	50
1993	108	45	42
Totals	379	159	42

Source: adapted from Delbeke et al (1995)

The analysis of the Flemish results also indicated the high level of steroids being taken (sometimes over twenty times the therapeutic dose), and the tendency towards multiple drug use. Abusers often took a number of different steroids at the same time, with stimulants and diuretics also found in some samples: the former probably for their appetite-suppressing properties and the latter in order to achieve the "sculpted" look desired for competition.

Among body builders there is a clear association between the use of anabolic steroids and psychological disorders associated with distorted body images.[2] A study of 108 body builders (fifty-five steroid users and fifty-three non-users) found cases of two types of body image disorders. A total of 28% of the total sample reported a history of anorexia nervosa (the norm for American males is 0.02%) and 8.3%, including two of those who had reported a history of anorexia nervosa, reported reverse anorexia, a condition in which they perceive themselves to be weak and small even though they are large and muscular. All the reverse anorexia cases were found among the steroid users and according to the responses to the structured interviews contributed to their decision to start taking steroids.[3] A study of the relationship

1. Delbeke, F.T, Desmet, M. & Debackere, M., "The Abuse of Doping Agents in Competing Body Builders in Flanders (1988-1993)", *International Journal of Sports Medicine*, Vol. 16, pp. 66-70 (1995).
2. This section draws on the review of recent research into steroid use by Bahrke, M.S., Yesalis, C.E. III & Wright, J.E., "Psychological and Behavioural Effects of Endogenous Testosterone and Anabolic-Androgenic Steroids, An Update", *Sports Medicine*, Vol. 22.6, pp. 367-390 (1996).
3. Pope, H., Katz, D. & Hudson, J.,"Anorexia Nervosa and ' Reverse Anorexia' Among 108 Male Bodybuilders", *Comprehensive Psychiatry*, Vol. 34.6, pp. 406-9 (1993).

between steroid use and self-perception of the body.[1] In their study they compared a group of body builders with groups of runners and martial artists and found that the body builders had the highest levels of self-reported steroid use and also the strongest expressions of dissatisfaction with their bodies. With the caveat that the evidence of steroid use is based on self-reporting, the study found that 44.2% of body builders used steroids, but only 2.1% of runners and no martial artists used the drugs. Not only did body builders provide stronger expressions of body dissatisfaction, but they also possessed lower levels of self-esteem and personal effectiveness. Their conclusions supported earlier studies that suggested that men who perceive themselves as underweight may become involved in body building and the use of anabolic steroids in order to achieve an exaggerated "hypermorphic" look. Porcerelli and Sandler measured the degree of narcissism among a group of weightlifters and body builders, some of whom used steroids and found that the steroid-using group scored much higher on a scale measuring pathological narcissism.[2] The diagnostic criteria for narcissistic personality disorder include a "grandiose sense of self-importance; pre-occupation with fantasies of omnipotence and omniscience; susceptibility to feelings of rage, shame, humiliation and emptiness; a sense of entitlement; exploitativeness; and a lack of empathy".[3] Whether it is immersion in the culture of body building that predisposes participants to develop low self-esteem and take steroids or whether those with low self-esteem are predisposed to participate in body building and take steroids is unclear.

Drugs and leisure sports

The theme of low self-esteem is also part of the discussion surrounding drug use, over-training and obsessive behaviour among those who participate in activities which are on the fringe of competitive sport, such as aerobics and keep fit. In an analysis of a series of surveys of steroid use in the United States, it was found that over one million people were spending more than US$100 million per year on steroids, with almost half the total number of users being under 25-years-old. In addition, it is estimated that between 4% and 11% of male adolescents and 0.5% and 2.9% of female adolescents had taken steroids at some time.[4] While many of those using steroids were involved in competitive sport, a substantial proportion were not and did not aspire to participate in competitive sport. Some 20% of recreational body builders admitted using steroids.

1. Blouin, A. & Goldfield, G. "Body Image and Steroid Use in Male Bodybuilders", *International Journal of Eating Disorders*, Vol. 18.2, pp. 159-65 (1995).
2. Porcerelli, J. & Sandler, B. "Narcissism and Empathy in Steroid Users", *American Journal of Psychiatry*, Vol. 152.11, pp. 1672-4 (1995).
3. bid., p. 1672.
4. Middleman, A.B. & DuRant, R.H. "Anabolic Steroid Use and Associated Health Risk Behaviours", *Sports Medicine*, Vol. 21.4 (1996).

Clearly there is a range of motives prompting the use of steroids and other ergogenic drugs among those involved in fringe sports activities. Among the young there is some evidence of strong pressure to conform to peer group expectations. Steroids, for example, are simply added to the list of currently fashionable recreational drugs such as ecstasy, marijuana and amphetamines. In addition, there are clear pressures arising from low self-esteem and the assumption that self-esteem can be enhanced if one's physique is closer to some ideal of masculinity or femininity. Whereas in the past it was assumed that the patriarchal character of society put intense pressure on women to attempt to shape their bodies to conform to male expectations, there is evidence that an increasing number of males feel under much the same pressure to shape their bodies to fit a socially constructed ideal.

As indicated in Figure 4.2, the various drug-taking communities both within sport and outside overlap, with athletes moving between elite competitive and non-elite competitive sport and between sport and non-sport communities. It is therefore not possible to treat drug abuse by athletes as a discrete phenomenon when one is examining policy options. Consequently, it is important to review, if only briefly, the attempts that have been made to control drug abuse in wider society in order to identify policy options that might inform the development of the anti-doping effort in sport.

Drug use and abuse beyond sport

Any attempt to outline and analyse a policy issue as complex as that concerned with drug abuse is beset with problems, not least of which is the enormous number of organisations with a direct or indirect interest in the issue and the dynamic nature of both problems and policies. In order to identify the key issues and factors that will be relevant to the discussion of current anti-doping policy in sport, it is necessary to adopt some fairly drastic simplifying measures. Some of the detail and nuances of the issue will be blurred but the reward is a sharper focus on the key aspects of the course of problem definition and policy response.

Drug use – whose problem?

Problems are rarely if ever self-evident. What might appear to one person as a pressing public problem demanding urgent intervention might appear to someone else as a private matter with which governments should avoid getting involved. At different times and in different societies issues as diverse as domestic violence, poverty, diet and youth homelessness were all considered to be private and personal issues rather than public problems. The same is true of the history of social and recreational drug use. In almost all countries over the last hundred years or so, there has been a shift in perception of drug use from a matter of personal choice and consequence to, on occasion, a matter of urgent government priority. Even today there is, in a number of countries, a recurring debate about whether drug use should be a matter for such intense government policy concern.

In many countries it is only a comparatively short time ago that opiates and cocaine were deemed to be relatively harmless and were routinely present in many medicines and tonics for both adults and children. Even well into the twentieth century there have been frequent calls for the decriminalisation of cocaine and heroin. Yet today the opiates and cocaine are perceived as dangerous "hard" drugs with few if any positive features. The history of the definition of drug use as a public problem obviously varies from one country to another, both in terms of the substances considered to be problematic and also in terms of the groups and organisations that were involved in the debate over drug use. In most industrialised and many developing countries there is currently a broad agreement that the opiates, marijuana, cocaine and hallucogenics should be illegal, while alcohol and tobacco should not. One of the problems encountered in the policy response to contemporary drug use is the practice of grouping a wide and varied range of substances under the heading of "drugs", a catch-all simplification that encourages misplaced efforts to devise uniform policies for a broad array of diverse problems.[1]

In explaining how decisions are taken about which drugs to target, it is important to take account of the variety of ways in which the problem of drug abuse can be framed. In some countries the debate on drug abuse has been stimulated and subsequently dominated by health care professionals, and in other countries the motivation for policy making has come from groups, such as churches and political parties, concerned with moral standards in society. Other definitions of the problem of drug use have come from those with a primary focus on the law-and-order aspects of the issue, or a concern with the impact of the drugs trade on international relations and political stability. Perceptions of the issue are crucial in determining the organisations that become involved in selecting policy solutions. However, it is not simply the case that perceptions of the issue of drug use vary between countries; they also differ over time in the same country. In Britain, for example, the perception of heroin addiction has changed over the forty-year period between the mid 1920s and the mid 1960s from "an individualised pathology affecting unfortunates, to a socially infectious condition, needing to be controlled",[2] with influence over policy moving from doctors, who were able to use their professional judgement to decide whether to prescribe heroin to addicts, to politicians, police and the courts, who ushered in a more punitive policy which saw the drug user ceasing to be a victim and becoming a villain.

1. Smith, P.H., "The Political Economy of Drugs, Conceptual Issues and Policy Options", in Smith, P.H., *Drug Policy in the Americas*, Boulder, Col., Westview Press (1992).
2. Lart, R. "British Medical Perception from Rolleston to Brain, Changing Images of the Addict and Addiction", *International Journal on Drug Policy*, Vol. 3, p. 19 (1992).

A similar inconsistency in attitudes and policy can be found in the United States where attitudes towards drug use have changed radically more than once over the last hundred years. Hailed as a wonder drug in the late nineteenth century, cocaine, for example, was rapidly demonised in the early years of the present century as a threat to the fabric of society and a danger to personal morality. Although the emphasis remained on care and cure, limitations were gradually placed on the freedom of doctors to prescribe cocaine or heroin. Gradually, during the 1920s, care and cure and the broadly welfare-based definition of the problem was replaced by criminalisation and ostracism. But even this redefinition was temporary as the cycle of liberalism followed by intolerance was repeated in the 1960s. The position on drug use adopted by most European communist governments was, at worst, simply denial that a problem existed. Given the prevalence of rhetoric which portrayed drug use as a product of capitalist societies and symptomatic of their decadence, it was extremely difficult for these countries to acknowledge that they too had a drug abuse problem.[1]

Doping in sport: athletes as victims or villains

Many of the dilemmas faced by those engaged in attempting to reduce recreational drug use have parallels in the development of anti-doping policy in sport. As with recreational anti-drugs policy, the anti-doping policy in sport has been variously conceptualised as a moral issue (one of cheating) and a health issue. There has also been considerable debate as to whether the issue is a private matter to be left to sports organisations or a matter of public policy which consequently involves governments. Finally, the definition of the problem takes place at both the international level and at the level of individual countries. There is still considerable tension between sports organisations, particularly the IOC and the major federations, over the issue of policy leadership and issue definition, and also tension between governmental and sports bodies over their respective roles and responsibilities in anti-doping policy.

The dominant definition of the issue of doping in sport remains, not surprisingly, that it is cheating. Underpinning this definition is a perception of the athlete as a rational person who is capable of making informed choices and who is aware of the unethical nature of doping. The decision to take drugs consequently makes the athlete a villain. Such a view, as will be shown below, led to policies that stressed detection and punishment. More recently, greater stress has been placed on the definition of doping as a serious health risk with athletes being, at least, partly ignorant of the medium and long-term consequences of their actions for their own health. The broadening of the definition of the problem is due, in part, to the increasing role of scientists, doctors and psychologists within sport and the different perspectives they bring to the problem. Although health concerns are still of secondary

1. Inciardi, J., "Drug Abuse in the Georgian SSR", *Journal of Psychoactive Drugs*, Vol. 19.4, pp. 329-34 (1987).

importance to ethics as the basis for current policy, there has been a growing emphasis placed on education and information.

The mix of definitions of the problem of doping is reflected in the list of banned substances and practices produced by the IOC. The evolution of the list has been shaped by the various interested parties concerned with doping such as doctors, sports administrators, scientists and, more recently, lawyers. Although each party will refer to a mix of criteria in attempting to shape the content of the IOC list, each will have, or at least should have, slightly different priorities. For sports doctors a prominent criterion should be the likelihood of damage to the athlete's health; for scientists the existence of a reliable test for a particular drug should be a central criterion; for sports administrators the ergogenic potential will be crucial, but there will also be a concern to protect the public image of sport; while for lawyers the reliability of testing methods and the probity of the testing process will be their main concerns.

The composition of the IOC list is the product of the interplay of the various interests concerned with anti-doping policy and as such is a regularly negotiated compromise. Where scientists might apply a strict interpretation of the ergogenic effect in order to determine inclusion, others, such as sports administrators concerned with the public image of sport, have pressed for the retention of drugs such as marijuana which have a negative public image but have, at best, a doubtful ergogenic value. A similar compromise exists between those who support a ban on narcotic analgesics such as cocaine, but who also support the permissibility of the administration of local anaesthetics, and those who consider that the latter should be banned because they too confer an advantage through the alteration of the athlete's natural state. In summary, the IOC list mirrors the balance of influence among those with an involvement in anti-doping policy at a particular time and is a compromise that reflects the current mix of science, morality and administrative pragmatism.

Setting objectives

The lack of a stable consensus in defining the problem of recreational drug use is complemented by a similar lack of consensus over the objectives to be achieved through the anti-drugs policy. Acknowledging that objectives will vary according to the type of drug being considered, there is still significant variation in objectives even for the same class of drug. At differing times the objectives have been set in terms of containment, control, treatment and elimination with the emphasis often reflecting whether priority is being given to the eradication of supply or the decrease in demand. In practice governments often adopted policy objectives which combined a dual focus on supply and demand. Finally, it is important to note that in some countries the "drug problem" has been subsumed by a concern with the levels of crime associated with the use of "hard drugs". As a result the primary emphasis has been placed on the elimination or, at least, the reduction of drug-related crime with the reduction in drug use itself relegated to a secondary outcome.

In the United States, for example, the emphasis has generally been on the development of policies designed to reduce supply rather than decrease demand, on the assumption that without a steady supply the demand for drugs will wither. Where and when the emphasis has been placed on addressing the demand for drugs, objectives have ranged from complete elimination through containment or management to tolerance. Sweden is an example of a country seeking to achieve elimination and consequently where "no distinction [is] made between soft and hard drugs, criminal law is invoked punitively, prevention, treatment and rehabilitation are emphasised and compulsory care can be imposed".[1] A similar set of objectives was dominant in Germany until recently and was reflected in a rejection of methadone maintenance programmes in preference for policies that sought to cut drug users off from their supply. By contrast, Switzerland, Denmark and Holland have tended to favour policies described as "harm minimisation" or "problem management". In general, countries have tended to oscillate between aiming for elimination and containment with tolerance being debated as a possible objective but one which is rarely adopted.

Given the ambiguity and variability over time of the policy objectives related to recreational drug use, are those for doping in sport any clearer? Bearing in mind the involvement of governments, the IOC, sports federations and domestic governing bodies of sport, is there a consensus regarding policy objectives? With only marginal exceptions, the primary objective of current policy has been to reduce demand rather than attempt to reduce supply. In some respects this is a pragmatic objective because of the fact that many banned substances are legal and relatively easily available and also have multiple sources of supply. However, there are some substances, such as synthetic human growth hormone and synthetic erythropoietin, both of which are tightly controlled, that have only a small number of suppliers and which therefore lend themselves to policies designed to achieve an attenuation of supply. Similarly, there are some substances whose successful administration is extremely difficult, if not hazardous, without professional assistance. Although restricting supply to athletes is difficult there appears to have been little consideration of this as a possible objective.

There is also a high level of ambiguity regarding the scope of anti-doping policy. The IOC is concerned with the elimination of doping at competitions organised under the auspices of the Olympic movement in order to be able to ensure the probity of results. The international federations vary considerably in the application of anti-doping policy, with some limiting testing to established elite athletes, others to elite and near elite, and still others

---

1. Ruggiero & South, p. 36, op. cit. (1995).

extending coverage to include juniors and veterans. While some governments see doping in sport as part of a broader anti-drugs policy, others tend to treat doping as a minor problem best left to sports authorities. Thus, doping in fringe sports such as body building is often ignored as it falls outside the mainstream concerns of sports organisations and the government. Overall there is little evidence of consistency and stability regarding objectives of sports anti-doping policy, although the level of dissension is far lower than in previous years and there is at least the basis for discussions about closer policy harmonisation.

Despite the progress that has been made in recent years towards harmonisation of objectives over the last thirty years or so, governments have demonstrated a wide variety of motives and levels of commitment to anti-doping. Despite public statements condemning doping, it is accepted that the governments of a number of the most prominent sporting countries were systematically undermining anti-doping efforts, while a further group of countries were allowing policy momentum to dissipate through lack of support.

The drive for anti-doping policy harmonisation currently being led by the Council of Europe and the IOC has sharpened many of the concerns regarding objectives. Among the objectives that need to be clarified are those relating to the boundary between ergogenic and recreational drug use, between treating the drug-using athlete as a villain who requires punishment or treating him/her as a victim who requires support, counselling and medical help, and between the burden of responsibility shouldered by the athlete and by members of his/her entourage. In addition, it must be asked whether the ultimate objective is the complete elimination of drug use in all sport, in certain sports, or only in sport at certain levels. Is the objective elimination or simply the containment of the extent of drug use? If, however, the objective is complete elimination then what level of commitment and resource allocation would be required for its achievement? Would the necessary commitment and resources be made available and where they would come from?

Selecting policy instruments

At some stage in the process of drawing up policy, decisions will have to be made about the most appropriate instruments (solution) to achieve the desired objectives. Although logically the setting of objectives should precede the identification of policy instruments this is not always the case as, in practice, solutions, currently being applied to other problems, may be applied to new problems. There are many examples of this practice in relation to drugs policy, indeed in most countries anti-drug strategies are typified by a high degree of uniformity in policy response with there being, for example, few significant illustrations of countries seeking to tailor policies to particular categories of drug user or particular drugs.

Over the years a wide range of policy solutions have been developed and applied to aspects of the recreational drug problem. Policy solutions may be categorised in a number of ways, such as according to the objective, but it is frequently the case that the same solution may be used to achieve a variety of objectives. It is more useful to categorise policy solutions in terms of the extent to which they rely on extrinsic or intrinsic instruments, with incentives or penalties being examples of the former and changes in attitudes being an example of the latter. Table 4.2 provides a simple schematic presentation of combinations of policy instrument with particular causes of non-compliance. First of all, judgements have to be made about the causes of non-compliance with objectives. For some, the cause of non-compliance might be ignorance or inability to comply, while for others the cause may lie in a conscious decision not to comply. Each of these causes could be sub-divided: for example an inability to comply may be due to the level of intelligence of the individual, or the lack of a particular skill, such as speaking the language of the country in which he or she is resident, or it may be due to constraints imposed by others who consequently prevent compliance.

Table 4.2: Recreational drug use: the causes of non-compliance and the effectiveness of various policy instruments

	Policy instruments			
	Inducements		Constraints	
Cause of non-compliance	Rewards	Education/ information	Erection of barriers	Deterrents
Ignorance or incompetence	Negligible effect	Substantial effect	Moderate effect	Moderate effect
Inability to comply (lack of free will)	Negligible effect	Negligible effect	Negligible effect	Negligible effect
Conscious decision not to comply	Moderate effect	Negligible effect	Moderate effect	Moderate effect

Table 4.2 lists three main causes of non-compliance and suggests that these may be analysed in relation to the main distinctive types of policy instrument available to governments and to other authoritative bodies, such as sports federations and the IOC. The use of incentives or threats are among the most common instruments adopted by governments to attempt to ensure compliance, but the use of rewards (access to government resources such as finance, medical treatment, welfare services, etc.) is also common in anti-drugs policy. However, the limits of rewards are evident when related to the three causes of non-compliance identified in the table. Rewards are unlikely to be of much value where the impediments to compliance are the result of ignorance or some other barrier such as illiteracy, an inability to communicate in the

language of the host country or doubts over security of residence. By contrast rewards might be successful where the source of non-compliance lies in choice.

A policy solution that relies on education and information may be more successful than simple rewards in overcoming the causes of non-compliance and it is very common for the two to be used in combination. One would hope that ignorance could be overcome through the provision of information (such as the health warning provided on cigarette packets or clearer information regarding the side effects of steroids). Information coupled with rewards might also undermine the resolve of those who consciously resist compliance. However, information is unlikely to be of much value where the cause of non-compliance is a lack of free will.

Policy instruments actually deployed are often combinations of instruments, for example coupling rewards with information. It is also true that policy instruments that are based on inducements are frequently combined with threats or constraints. For example, barriers may be erected to make the targeted behaviour more difficult to undertake. Barriers may be of various types including physical (fences or trenches at football grounds to prevent pitch invasions), psychological (street cameras in "red light" areas), and bureaucratic (high levels of tax on tobacco). Stronger constraints may come in the form of deterrents such as threats of exclusion, imprisonment or fines. The success of policy instruments derived from constraints is also affected by the cause of non-compliance. Constraints are not going to be of much value where the basis of non-compliance is ignorance or a lack of choice or free will. Threats and other constraints may, however, be more successful where non-compliance is the result of a conscious decision to break a regulation or law.

At the domestic level, policy instruments designed to reduce demand frequently rely on combinations of inducements and constraints. In the past the emphasis has tended to be on increasing the cost to the drug user of obtaining drugs by, for example, an intensive arrest and prosecution policy which imposes on the user the cost of punishment. More recently there has been a trend away from a reliance on constraints and a more sympathetic attitude towards policy instruments aimed at reducing demand by the treatment of existing users, for example with heroin substitute, and education of potential users to avoid drugs.[1] The policy instrument is partly an inducement, as care and a steady supply of the heroin substitute are offered as a reward for compliance.

In addition to strategies targeted at established drug users, there are also examples of strategies aimed at preventing the non-user or occasional user becoming an established user. Where the policy objective is drug prevention (in other words a reduction in demand), the policy instrument is usually focused on the provision of information and education about the dangers of

1. Hough, M., *Problem Drug use and Criminal Justice*, London, Home Office Drug Prevention Initiative (1996).

drug misuse and may be targeted at potential users, their peer group and their parents and teachers.[1]

The possible combinations of policy instruments is vast and the examples given above are designed to illustrate current policy and, more importantly, to provide a point of comparison when considering current anti-doping policy in sport. Table 4.3 adopts the same framework for exploring the relationship between causes of non-compliance with anti-doping regulations and policy instruments. The most obvious cause of non-compliance is a conscious decision to seek a competitive advantage through the use of drugs, but it is not the only cause. For example, there are plenty of examples of athletes who would claim that they had little option but to take drugs due to the character of the political regime under which they lived. However, the debate about the limits imposed by others on an athlete's free will is a highly controversial basis for non-compliance and one that is examined in detail in the next chapter. In contrast, ignorance or lack of competence is a more plausible basis for non-compliance. There are many examples of athletes claiming ignorance of the chemical properties of medicines and given the complexity of the current IOC list it is probably unrealistic to expect every athlete to be familiar with the full list and its interpretation.

Table 4.3 : Doping in sport among adult athletes : causes of non-compliance and the likely effectiveness of policy instruments

Policy instruments				
	Inducements		Constraints	
Cause of non-compliance	Rewards	Education/ information	Erection of barriers	Deterrents
Ignorance or incompetence	Negligible effect	Substantial potential effect	Moderate effect	Negligible effect
Inability to comply (lack of free will)	Negligible effect	Negligible effect	Moderate effect	Negligible effect
Conscious decision not to comply	Moderate effect	Moderate effect	Moderate effect	Moderate effect

As regards the variety of instruments available to anti-doping authorities, the most commonly applied is the deterrent. Deterrents range from a life ban from competition, at one extreme, through fixed term bans to public warnings at the lenient end of the scale. Where drug users have broken the criminal law it is also possible that prison sentences might be imposed, although

---

1. Duke, K., MacGregor, S. & Smith, L., *Activating Local Networks, A Comparison of two Community Development Approaches to Drug Prevention*, London, Home Office Drug Prevention Initiative (1996).

there are few examples of custodial sentences. Deterrents are unlikely to be successful where the cause of non-compliance is either ignorance or incompetence. Deterrents are also likely to be of only limited value where athletes' choices regarding drug use are constrained, especially when the constraint is being imposed by the state. This policy instrument is therefore only likely to be effective when sports authorities are supported by the domestic government and where there is relatively easy access to athletes to conduct tests: in other words where the athlete is acting in an individual capacity (or with the support of only one or two others) in a country where both the governing bodies and government are supportive of the anti-doping policy.

The erection of barriers to inhibit drug use is an alternative policy instrument, but one that relies heavily on the co-operation of other groups or organisations that might not always share the same objectives as the supporters of anti-doping. For example, one could seek tighter control of the supply of drugs prepared by the pharmaceutical industry, especially those that are produced in relatively small quantities and which are mainly distributed through hospitals. However, how realistic is it to expect pharmaceutical companies to forgo the opportunity to expand the market for a particular drug? Ethics and profit are not always complementary. One might also expect doctors to constitute an effective barrier to the abuse of drugs, but such an expectation needs to be moderated by the knowledge that there are significant examples of doctors prescribing ergogenic drugs for athletes. For effective barriers to be erected, it probably would require government intervention to force greater control over supply on the part of the pharmaceutical companies and a greater willingness on the part of professional associations to interfere with the traditional autonomy of doctors to prescribe as they see fit. If barriers could be effectively established they would undoubtedly have a significant impact on the athlete's access to drugs, but the problems of erecting effective barriers are formidable and there are few examples, if any, of their success as policy instruments with regard to either recreational or sports drugs.

In many countries with an established anti-doping strategy, education is an increasingly important policy instrument. Targeted at both the junior and the adult athlete, educational programmes often seek to raise awareness of the health risks and the career risks associated with drug use, as well as promoting an appreciation of the ethical issues raised by doping. Where ignorance is the cause of drug use then obviously an educational programme is likely to be effective, but it is unlikely to have an impact on the other two causes of non-compliance.

Rewards have considerable potential to promote compliance. Many governments have rewarded athletes who they consider a model for their citizens with national honours and sports organisations have inducted athletes in "Halls of Fame". Although a clean record on drugs is not the sole criterion for a reward, it is often taken into account and may be effective with those athletes attracted by the long-term status that honours confer.

The IOC and most major international federations have, not surprisingly, relied on policy instruments which directly parallel those developed to combat recreational drug use. Among the most common instruments are threats of loss of eligibility to compete, often combined with programmes of education and information. But there are also examples, resulting from co-operation with governments, of attempts to restrict supply either through the tightening of control over access to drugs currently available "over the counter" in pharmacies or through attempts to limit the leakage of controlled drugs such as hGH into the black market. However, many questions remain including whether the balance of policy instruments is appropriate, and whether the mix of policy instruments varies to suit the type of drug use or drug user being targeted. In addition, there have been debates recently about whether the athlete is the proper target for anti-doping policy or whether members of the athlete's entourage, or indeed his/her national governing body, should be the proper focus for achieving compliance.

Monitoring implementation and measuring success

It is tempting to consider that, once agreement on objectives has been reached and policy instruments and implementing organisations have been selected, the bulk of the work involved in policy making is complete. This is not an accurate picture of the policy process. For a variety of reasons it is essential that ways are devised to measure the success of the selected policy instruments and agencies in achieving the desired objectives. However, what makes this task at times extremely problematic is that policy objectives are frequently unclear and subject to relatively rapid alteration.

One of the unavoidable dangers of using performance indicators is that frequently they are designed to measure outputs rather than outcomes. For example, in the campaign against social and recreational drug use claims of "success" are often based on increases in the volume of drugs intercepted at ports and borders, the arrest and successful prosecution of leading drug wholesalers, increases in the number of arrests of drug users and the ratification of anti-drug conventions promoted by international organisations. At best these measures are indirect and suggestive of progress but are highly unreliable as a guide to progress towards the central objective of reducing drug consumption and the number of drug users. For example, success in intercepting imported drugs might simply result in drug users switching to domestically produced alternatives, and increased arrest rates for drug users might simply transfer drug users from the streets to prisons where drug use is often extensive. In the context of the anti-doping campaign in sport, techniques for measuring progress towards policy objectives are poor, relying mainly, on trends in the number of positive test results.

Overall, the development of reliable performance measures for the assessment of the success of current anti-doping policy remains elusive and generally a low priority. A key problem is the reliability of the data currently collected. The numbers of positive results will be affected by various factors including the number of tests carried out, their distribution between sports, and the balance between in-competition and out-of-competition tests. Further, not all positive test results are deemed to be doping infractions. A second difficulty with the interpretation of doping records is that the decline in the number of positives for one type of drug might indicate success in anti-doping policy implementation but might, more plausibly, indicate an evolution in the drug culture, for example, away from amphetamines to steroids and, more recently, from steroids to testosterone, or greater sophistication among users in avoiding detection or, indeed, a shift to other less easily detected drugs. Finally, it remains difficult to identify reliable time series indicators of progress due to the rapidity with which the nature of the problem evolves. Not only do the range of available and preferred drugs continue to expand, but so too do the range of, and application of, testing procedures. As a result it is not possible to draw firm conclusions about the current level of policy success. Consequently, the repeated claims to be "winning the war on doping in sport" will continue to prompt scepticism rather than congratulations until a set of agreed benchmarks is established. Ironically, probably the best indicator of success is the decline in performance in some events at recent Olympic games. For example, there was a marked decline in performance in women's javelin, discus and shot-put following the introduction of out-of-competition testing in 1989.[1] Not only did the best performance of the year decline but so too did the average performance of the ten best athletes. In the shot, for example, the best performance in 1987 was over 22.5 metres, but between 1989 and 1993 no female athlete put the shot further than 22 metres and in 1996 no athlete exceeded 21 metres. A similar pattern is found in the javelin where no one has got within 4 metres of the 1988 world record and in 1996 the best throw was some 10.5 metres short of the record.

Policy review and modification

There are three developments that prompt a review of policy instruments: first, the failure of the policy to produce improvements in the selected measures of performance; second, the emergence of new dimensions to the target problem; and third, a redefinition of the problem. Given that problems are, at best, moving targets it is only to be expected that policy instruments will need to be regularly reviewed to ensure that they are still appropriate. In practice, however, it is common for policy to become fixed and to get progressively out of step with the problem it was intended to address. It is also

---

1. Franke & Berendonk, op. cit.

common for policy instruments to be subject to political competition as different interests attempt to affect the way in which the instrument is interpreted and applied. It is when examining the way in which policies are reviewed that the weaknesses of attempts to explain the policy process as a series of stages are most apparent.

Where debate is relatively open, the process of policy review may result in the decision to maintain the current policy. It may, however, result in the decision to replace the existing policy with one thought more suitable, that is policy succession. Alternative outcomes include the decision to modify the existing policy or indeed to terminate the policy.[1] The most common result is the decision to reconfigure the "ingredients" in the existing policy, for example, by altering the balance between constraints and inducements. In general, radical alterations to existing policy are often infrequent because interested bodies have too much credibility invested in particular policies. Within anti-drugs policy this is amply illustrated by the determination of many countries to resist the introduction of policies based on treatment, decriminalisation and reward to replace policies based on punishment of users and the interdiction of supply. With regard to current anti-doping policy it might seem premature to discuss policy review and modification when many would argue that the policy is still being established. However, one feature of sport drug abuse is the pace at which the problem evolves, due to both the advent of new drugs and to the emergence of new problems such as the increasing frequency of legal challenges to federation decisions. The current concern with policy harmonisation is providing an important opportunity for policy review and refinement.

Conclusion

Although doping in sport has a number of distinctive features, the key conclusion of this chapter is that it is not possible to isolate the problem of doping in sport from the wider issues of related drug abuse in society, no more than it is possible to isolate sportsmen and women from drug abuse in wider society. There is also a deep interconnection between domestic and international policy making and the wide range of organisations that are active in the policy process. A similar range of organisations are involved in combating drug abuse in sport and successful policy implementation relies on a co-ordinated strategy functioning at both the international and the domestic levels. Where drug abuse in sport differs from recreational drug abuse is that the organisational source of policy momentum in sport lies more securely at the international level, with the IOC and the IAAF in particular. Nevertheless, the sport anti-doping policy is just as vulnerable as recreational drug abuse policy to being undermined by weak support at the domestic level.

---

1. See Hogwood, B. & Peters, B.G., *Policy Dynamics*, Brighton, Wheatsheaf Books (1983).

Sport also shares similarities with recreational drug abuse insofar as the character of the problem being addressed is not static. The evolution of the issue has been marked by change, not only in terms of the drugs considered to be the most serious challenge to the integrity of competitive sport, but also in terms of the sports most at risk from corruption through drug use. It is not surprising that the sports and governmental bodies at the heart of the anti-doping strategy have utilised a range of policy instruments over the last twenty years: however, most of them have been adaptations of existing instruments used to tackle problems of recreational drug abuse. This brief review of the way in which the issue of drug abuse has been defined and redefined illustrates not only the shifting nature of the definition of social problems, but also the variety of organisations and interests involved in attempting to influence the process of definition. Doctors, welfare professionals, politicians, courts and the police are only some of the more prominent interests involved in shaping policy at the domestic level. Although it is possible to characterise drug abuse as a personal or community problem, it is increasingly accepted that it is located within a global context of production and supply. When account is taken of the international dimension of problem definition, it would be necessary to examine the contribution of individual governments, international police networks and international government organisations such as the United Nations and the European Union.

Chapter 5

Defining the problem: the ethics of doping

Doping, it is often argued, is anathema in sport because it is unfair. If further defence is required then it may also be argued that doping in sport is "cheating, plain and simple",[1] is dangerous to the health of the athlete, is harmful to the image of the activity and may deter sponsors, or is a poor example to set to younger, aspiring athletes. If these justifications fail to impress then the circular argument is relied upon that doping is a breach of governing body rules. As will be shown below, all these arguments have a certain plausibility but none is, by itself, capable of providing a sufficiently strong underpinning for the enormous investment of resources currently devoted to the anti-doping strategy.

Until a satisfactory answer can be given to the question "Why oppose doping?", it is not possible to define with sufficient clarity the problem that the sporting and governmental authorities are trying to tackle nor is it possible to defend anti-doping policy with confidence. Moreover, the policy instruments selected will, to a very large extent, be determined by the formulation of the basis on which doping is opposed. Quite simply, if the primary objection is that doping damages the health of athletes, the policy instruments selected will be very different from those chosen if the problem is formulated solely as a breach of sporting ethics.

The central focus of this chapter is on an examination of the basis on which doping in sport may be opposed. A second aspect of the issue of doping in sport, namely how sporting and other organisations define the problem they are addressing, forms the basis of Chapter 6 which examines current anti-doping policy.

In most recent discussions of doping there are a limited number of recurring justifications for opposing doping. In the concluding chapter of his report into drug abuse by athletes in Canada, Justice Dubin quoted from the Olympic Charter which states that "They [the Olympic Games] unite Olympic competitors of all countries in fair and equal competition". He then proceeded to castigate Canadian athletes who have not lived up to this ideal and who "resorted to performance-enhancing drugs and other banned practices, thereby gaining an unfair advantage over those who did not do so (...) Those who have cheated have threatened the very future of sport and tarnished its reputation (...) They have also unfairly cast a cloud of suspicion over the

---

1. Voy, R. *Drugs, Sport and Politics, The Inside Story About Drug Use in Sport and its Political Cover-up*, Champaign, Ill., Leisure Press (1991).

majority of athletes, who abide by the rules, and have threatened their future financial support from governments, corporations, and the general public".[1] A similar view is expressed by members of the Australian Senate Committee investigation into drugs in sport. Following an extensive discussion of the possible reasons for opposing drug use, the committee concludes:

> "The committee takes the view that performance-enhancing drugs should be banned because they can potentially damage the health of those taking them, whether they are elite athletes who stand the risk of being detected using them, or the recreational sportsperson who is unlikely ever to be tested. They should be banned also because anyone using them is trying to gain an unfair advantages over those athletes who wish to maintain normal health. They are cheating, because their use is against the rules of the sporting federations."[2]

These three reflections on the rationale for opposing doping in sport have much in common. For the IOC, the essential reason for attempting to ban doping is a wish to protect fair and equal competition. That doping should be opposed because it introduces inequality and unfairness into sport is a view shared by Justice Dubin who refers to the desire to seek an unfair advantage as cheating, but also adds that doping should be opposed for the additional reason that doping might undermine the financial viability of sport due to the withdrawal of government and corporate support. Not only is doping cheating, it is also inimical to the security of the resource base of the activity. The Australian Senate Committee, like Dubin and the IOC, bases its condemnation of doping on the grounds that it is cheating, but also adds that the potential health risks provide a further justification for banning drugs. In summary, the rationale for the investment of extensive resources in developing an anti-doping strategy is first, that it is potentially injurious to the athlete's health, second that doping is unfair, and third that it might undermine the credibility of sport in the eyes of external bodies or interests including government, corporations and the general public. It is important to note not only the variety of possible justifications but the specific focus of each justification. The first, harm to the athlete, takes the individual as its focus, the second, unfairness, directs attention to the sports community or co-competitors of the drug-user, while the third is framed in terms of abstract notions of the ideals of sport.

Athlete's rights and responsibilities

It is worth emphasising at this stage in the discussion the importance of the tension between these three justifications and particularly the potential for

---

1. Dubin Report (1990), "Commission of Enquiry into the use of Drugs and Banned Practices Intended to Increase Athletic Performance", Commissioner, Honourable C.L. Dubin, Ottawa, Canadian Government Publishing Centre, p. 517.
2. Commonwealth of Australia (1989), "Drugs in Sport", An Interim Report of the Senate Standing Committee on Environment, Recreation and the Arts, Canberra, Commonwealth of Australia, p. 60.

conflict between a rationale built upon the rights (and occasionally the obligations) of the individual and the interests of the sporting community. For many, sport represents an embodiment of the virtues of individualism and a profound metaphor for the political value of liberal individualism where the rights of the individual are seen as prior to the interests of society or community. Sportsmen and women, through their hard work, risk-taking and dedication seek to achieve success in competition. Such a strong liberal tradition, especially in the United States, makes many wary of sanctioning any further intrusion upon the rights of individual athletes. The current growth in commercialism in sport provides further justification for those critical of current anti-doping policy who argue that athletes' rights to earn a living must be protected. However, the contrary view stresses the obligations of the sportsman or woman to other athletes, arguing that sporting competition is not an isolated activity and is not possible without a community of athletes to compete against.

Many of the arguments about anti-doping policy share a common concern to see the athlete as part of a sports community, a view which recognises their rights but also accepts that they have responsibilities as well. The tension between the right of the individual to pursue his/her own interests as long as they do not interfere with the freedom of others taps deeply held values in many countries. Opponents of current anti-doping policy frequently justify, or at least strengthen, their opposition by emphasising the importance of limiting infringements of the rights of the individual athlete while the proponents of current policy emphasise that athletic activity, by its very nature, is a community enterprise. As will become clear, the contemporary debate on the justification for an anti-doping policy is sharply focused around questions of individual rights, community interests and ascribed ideals of sport and is a key theme that will be returned to more explicitly in the concluding discussion.

When the issue of drug use by athletes is being considered, it is understandable that the focus tends to be on exemplar drugs, most commonly anabolic steroids which, using Lavin's terminology, may be described as additive insofar as they "let users reach performance levels exceeding what they might otherwise reach when healthy".[1] The central focus of this chapter is on the use of additive drugs but it is important to bear in mind that other categories of drug exist which cannot always be treated in the same way. Apart from additive drugs there are those which are restorative in character and which are either designed or intended to restore an injured athlete to "normal" functioning. In addition, there are also drugs that have been taken by athletes but which have no proven ergogenic properties and which are primarily recreational.

---

1. Lavin, M. "Sports and Drugs, Are the Current Bans Justified?", *Journal of the Philosophy of Sport*, Vol. XIV, pp. 34-43 (1987).

Doping is unfair

Although there are other justifications for the current anti-doping policy, it is appropriate that the discussion should begin with an evaluation of the most commonly offered rationale, namely that doping is unfair. While unfairness is the most common justification, it is also one of the most problematic. Simply to assert that doping confers an advantage is an insufficient justification for banning doping as it can be powerfully argued that sport is all about seeking an advantage over other competitors. Much of the strength of this argument hinges on the distinction between a fair and an unfair advantage. Sportsmen and women will spend much of their time seeking an advantage over others through the development of improved training techniques, diet and equipment. As Black and Pape argue "Athletes turn to every possible device to improve their performance, including coaching, high-altitude training, videos, amino acids, special diets, vitamins, and drugs".[1] In addition, athletes start with differing physiological and psychological attributes and profiles which will give some an advantage over others. As a result, it is not a cause of adverse comment when we find that one boxer has more stamina or a longer reach than his opponent or when one footballer has a better sense of balance than another, or when one netball player is taller than her opponent. In general, advantages conferred by nature do not lead to accusations of unfairness. The only exception, and then only partial, is where the disparity in natural endowments is so marked that the quality of the contest is devalued or undermined.

In some sports, therefore, such as boxing, wrestling, judo and weightlifting, the international federations segregate competition by weight. There are also many sports that segregate by sex or age for similar reasons. However, the rationale for the creation of weight divisions, for example, is not based on a perception of a weight advantage as a form of cheating but due to a desire to preserve what they consider to be the essential nature of the contest; in the case of boxing, the balance of strength, stamina and skill that prevents a one-sided contest. Yet even this response to unevenness in natural abilities and endowments between athletes is not consistently applied. In tennis, for example, there is no complaint when the number one seed is drawn against an opponent a hundred or so places below him/her in the ranking table. Leaving aside the degree of inconsistency in the application of the practice of segregation in sporting contest, it does raise the intriguing prospect that one solution to the problem of drug use is to segregate according to drug use. Some weightlifting and body building contests already offer drug-free competitions alongside "open" competitions. Natural advantage is not considered to be an unfair advantage, although rules might be adjusted to take account of natural endowments. However, it is not sufficient to argue that

---

1. Black, T. & Pape, A., "The Ban on Drugs in Sport, The Solution or the Problem?", *Journal of Sport and Social Issues*, Vol. 21.1, pp. 83-92, (1997).

the dividing line between what is ethical and what is not can be drawn between natural and unnatural advantages for, as will be shown, not all unnatural advantages are considered to be in the same category as doping. It is also the case that the current generation of new drugs contain a number which are natural (or naturally occurring if not naturally achieved) such as blood doping and enhanced levels of testosterone.

Seeking "the edge"

It has already been suggested that sport is predicated on the search for an advantage or an "edge" over one's rivals and that exploiting one's natural advantages for example through more effective or rigorous training is applauded rather than frowned upon. As Fost observes, "The mere seeking of an advantage is not implicitly unfair, nor is the gaining of an advantage implicitly unfair.[1] The question of the boundary between what is fair and what is unfair is blurred, albeit slightly, when account is taken of advantages whose source is external to the athlete. For example, while most people would consider the pursuit of an intensive and rigorous training schedule as reflecting many of the virtues of sport such as dedication and application, would the same response be generated if the improvement in performance had been due to the outcome of an elaborate and expensive computer analysis of the athlete's technique? In this situation one might argue that the advantage accruing to the athlete is still the product of his/her effort and dedication. But supposing the advantage was the result of a swimmer wearing swimwear with ultra-low water resistance, a cyclist riding a cycle that incorporated state of the art design and materials, a pole-vaulter using a pole with additional spring and strength, or a Formula One racing driver whose car has the best engine and best engineers? In all these cases the source of the advantage is, like anabolic steroids for example, external to the athlete, but, unlike anabolic steroids, the response of sports authorities is less clear cut. Perry in his discussion of the ethics of blood doping suggests a test for the permissibility of an external, or in his words supplementary, advantage.[2] He suggests that if an enhanced performance due to supplementation is to be accepted, it must fulfil at least one of two key functions: to eliminate a deleterious effect (for example, a new shoe design may reduce the risk of ankle injury), or to remove a barrier to improved performance (allowing the use of synthetic running surfaces or the use of running spikes). In addition, one might add a third criterion, namely that advantages gained through supplementation must also be generally available. Applying Perry's criteria, it would not be possible to argue that drugs such as steroids or human growth

---

1. Fost, N.C. "Ethical and Social Issues in Anti-doping Strategies in Sport", in Landry, F., Landry, M. & Yerles, M. (eds.) *Sport ... The Third Millennium*, Sainte-Foy, Les Presses de l' Université de Laval (1991).
2. Perry, C. "Blood Doping and Athletic Competition", *The International Journal of Applied Philosophy*, Vol. 1.3, pp. 39-45 (1983).

hormone "eliminate a deleterious effect", as most agree that they may cause deleterious side effects (to the user if not to the quality of the sporting spectacle). It is doubtful whether it is possible to sustain the argument that any drugs eliminate a deleterious effect although there may be a case to be made with regard to restorative as opposed to additive drugs. Perry's second criterion, along with the third, would provide a justification for drug use if it is accepted that some drugs do indeed provide an ergogenic advantage and that drugs are generally available.

Differential access

When the American pole-vaulter, Bob Seagren, sought to use a fibreglass pole at the 1972 Olympic Games, its use was prohibited until the new pole became more widely available. However, the rationale for the prohibition was that differential access to the new pole was unfair, not that the pole itself was illegitimate. Similarly, when the Németh javelin with its improved aerodynamics was introduced, it provided a distinct advantage over the more conventional Sandvik javelin until the former was banned in late 1991.[1] Yet there are many examples of advances in equipment that have not led to bans, either temporary or permanent. The use by American swimmers of low-friction swimsuits, the Lotus-designed cycle and the use of aerodynamically designed helmets, skis and ski-sticks have all, at various times, conferred a generally acknowledged advantage upon those able to gain initial access. The response by sports authorities to unnatural advantages which are clearly similar in their effect in competition is far too inconsistent for a case against the use of drugs to be sustained simply on the basis of differential access. Moreover, there is a plausible case to be made that access to drugs is far from differential and that, at the elite level at least, access to drugs is reasonably uniform. Indeed, one could go much further and suggest that if the concern with the use of anabolic steroids and other ergogenic drugs is differential access then the balance of the argument favours removing the prohibition rather than attempting to enforce it. Black and Pape argue that the most appropriate response to the problem of differential access to the regularly produced advances in training, diet, etc., that give an athlete an edge over his or her competitors is to seek ways of speeding the process of diffusion. Policy, therefore, needs to be designed to ensure that the competitive edge conferred by a particular advance is reduced as rapidly as possible by making the advance available as widely as possible and as quickly as possible. As Black and Pape argue, "After the advantages gained by artificial devices are competed away, the most naturally gifted sportsperson will win".[2] The logic of this argument is that, far from maintaining fair competition, the (flawed) attempted imposition of a ban on drugs creates and magnifies unfairness in sport as only some athletes abide by the rules.

---

1. The main motive for banning the Németh javelin was the risk that the distances being achieved were outgrowing many arenas and becoming a danger to other athletes and also to the public.
2. Black, T. & Pape, A. (1997), op. cit., p. 85.

Black and Pape's argument has close parallels with the prohibition against "insider trading" on the stock market where traders seek an advantage over competitors through accessing information likely to affect share values before others and keeping such inside information secret until they secure their advantage. The response of regulators and legislators has not been to attempt to prohibit access to certain types of advantageous information (the equivalent of banned drugs in sport), but rather to ensure that information is made available as quickly as possible to all "players" in the market so as to "compete away" the advantage of selective access.[1]

One problem with the logic employed by Black and Pape is the assumption that the effect of free access to drugs would be to equalise advantage. As Gardner suggests, if unrestricted access to drugs were to be permitted, "inequalities would exist not just between users and non-users but among users".[2] Because athletes are unlikely to respond to drug use in the same way and to the same degree, inequalities would still remain. However, the inequalities arising from differential reactions to drugs would not necessarily give cause for complaint because it may be argued that the degree of benefit achieved is the result of natural differences in athletes' physiology and biochemistry. But a further problem would also remain, namely the fact that no matter how swiftly new drugs were made available someone would gain access first and be able to benefit first. If access by the first user coincided with a major tournament this might be sufficient to secure a very significant sporting and financial advantage. It would appear that each avenue that is taken in the pursuit of a secure basis for banning drugs on the grounds of fairness turns into a cul de sac of ambiguity or inconsistency, or worse still rebounds against the proponents of anti-doping policy and is used to challenge current policy.

One response to the ambivalence arising out of the discussion of differential access is to argue that rather than basing one's objection to an advantage which is external to the athlete on the extent of differential access one should rather ask whether the intention of the athlete was to keep the advantage secret. However, this is no more viable as a rationale for the banning of drugs than differential access as it is not possible to avoid the charge of inconsistency. Not only do many athletes closely guard the secrets of their training or dietary regimes but there are also examples of athletes who do not need to maintain the secrecy of their advantage because there are sufficient alternative and equally effective barriers to access such as cost and expertise. Hence, there are important advantages, such as training and dietary regimes, that are acknowledged to confer significant advantages but which do not prompt a significant ethical challenge although they do raise ethical concerns.

---

1. For a fuller examination of the ethics of insider trading, see Barry, N., *The Morality of Business Enterprise*, Aberdeen, Aberdeen University Press.
2. Gardner, R., "On Performance-enhancing Substances and the Unfair Advantage Argument", *Journal of the Philosophy of Sport*, Vol. XVI, pp. 59-73 (1989).

All a matter of perception?

It is possible that the acceptability of an advantage depends not on whether it is natural or unnatural, nor whether it is differentially available but rather on a perception of how the advantage is acquired. Advantages that accrue from location (it is an advantage to be a competitive skier living in Austria rather than in Holland), natural endowment (in soccer, Gianfranco Zola's sense of balance or Peter Schmichel's height), or practice (in cricket, Shane Warne's bowling action) are all significant but considered fair and indeed encouraged. A useful illustration of the importance of considering the process by which an advantage is gained is provided by attempts by bowlers in cricket to increase the variability of the flight of the ball. It is common, permissible and acceptable, for bowlers to polish one half of the ball so as to create conditions where the ball is more likely to spin due to the differential movement of air over the polished as opposed to the unpolished side. The existence of a polished and unpolished side also makes the bounce of the ball slightly more difficult to predict. An alternative way of creating the same effect is to score the unpolished side with the fingernail or even to attempt to lift the leather from the seam. While the polishing is acceptable scouring the leather is not and is considered to be ball tampering and treated as a serious breach of the rules of cricket by the governing body.

A second illustration of the importance of process is the methods used to improve the capacity of the blood to transport greater quantities of oxygen to the muscles. There are two common ways of making this improvement, the first is through blood doping and the second is through a prolonged period of high altitude training. While the former is condemned, the latter technique is acceptable. Interestingly, it does not seem to matter to the general public or those involved in sport if an advantage such as prolonged high altitude training is the result of greater wealth. It would appear that even if an advantage can be described as unfair, such as an unequal distribution of wealth, it does not mean that it will be perceived as being unacceptable. To take an exaggerated, but not implausible example, we might have a competition between two runners one of whom is born with an optimal physique, has wealthy supportive parents, benefits from the best coaches, trains in the relaxed atmosphere of a well-equipped university athletics club; the other is born with a physique that has potential to develop the necessary attributes, has an unsupportive family, works full-time and trains part-time at the local YMCA. If the two were to meet in competition and the former won it is unlikely that there would be any accusations of unfairness, although if the latter were victorious there might be some expressions of delight that the underdog had won through.

It is possible that acceptability depends on whether the advantage is either a natural endowment or has been earned through hard work and training. But the weaknesses of this suggestion are easily made apparent. How much effort is required to justify an advantage? Some athletes have to work much harder to secure their advantage than others: do the former have a stronger moral entitlement to the advantage than those who acquire the same advantage through a less onerous training regime? The inconsistencies in this argument do little to help in the search for a watertight basis for anti-doping policy.

Is the use of restorative drugs also unfair?

The preceding discussion has focused on the use of drugs whose function is additive, designed to give an athlete an advantage, rather than on those whose function is restorative. It is possible to argue that where an athlete is below his/her normal level of fitness, whether through illness or recovery from injury, the use of drugs simply to restore normal performance should not be subject to the same prohibition as the use of additive drugs. The argument is, at first sight, a powerful one. Athletes who have trained for a particular competition and then receive an injury whose effects can be nullified by the use of a drug can argue that they are not increasing their chances of success but simply maintaining their normal level of competitiveness. Leaving aside the complex problem of determining the athlete's "normal level of fitness" it is possible to treat restorative and additive drugs in the same way. At the heart of the issue is the way in which the concept of normality is being used. One way of defining an athlete's normal level of fitness is simply to say that it is that level of fitness possessed by the athlete at any particular time, and if they are ill the level of fitness they possess during their illness is their "normal" level. In other words, it cannot be accepted that an athlete is able to select their level of fitness at a particular time and claim that as their normal level of fitness. If this view is rejected then it would be possible, for example, for athletes who had sustained an injury which permanently reduced their capabilities to justify the use of drugs for the rest of their career as a way of restoring their pre-injury level of fitness.

If it is not possible to justify drug use where the objective is to restore an injured athlete to his/her normal level of fitness, then it should be even less acceptable to allow drug use where the athlete's "ill health" is due to decisions about training or diet. Hyland provides a good illustration of the dilemma by recounting the example of the American middle distance runner, Mary Decker Slaney. Due to her intensive training regime, Slaney's leg muscles had outgrown the sheath which contained them causing considerable pain. The problem was resolved by an operation that cut the muscle sheaths thereby relieving the pressure in her legs. At first glance the operation appears restorative in that it relieved the pain. On reflection one could argue that the pain she had been experiencing was a signal from her body that she had reached her limit of normal muscle growth and that the operation allowed abnormal growth and was therefore additive in character. As Hyland observes, Slaney could have "dealt with the problem just as well by slackening off on her training".[1]

---

1. Hyland, D.A., *Philosophy of Sport*, New York, Paragon House, p. 52.

Doping is a danger to the athlete's health

If a rationale for banning drugs constructed around fairness fails to provide the desired watertight basis for policy, an alternative is frequently sought in arguments framed in terms of the health of the athlete. As was made clear in the discussion of the effects and particularly the side effects of the variety of drugs banned by the IOC, there are some drugs where the weight of scientific opinion confirms that there are indeed clear deleterious effects arising from drug use but that there are also many banned substances where few if any significant side effects have (as yet) been identified. As a result, relying upon health-related arguments to provide a basis for anti-doping policy which is capable of covering all the drugs included on the IOC list is not possible. Nevertheless, it is worth exploring the health arguments in relation to those drugs, including steroids, amphetamines and human growth hormone, where scientific opinion warns of significant negative side effects. If it is assumed that the taking of some drugs poses substantial health risks to the athlete, the question remains as to whether this would provide a sufficient basis for prohibition.

For the purposes of the present discussion we will assume that we are considering drug use by adult athletes who are capable of making rational decisions. In relation to competent adults there is a general reluctance, especially in liberal democracies, to interfere with the individual's right to make choices about life-style even when those choices might contain a significant element of risk. This is especially evident in relation to current debates within the field of medical ethics, where there has been a determination in many European and North American countries to alter what has been characterised as an imbalance in the relationship between the doctor (professional) and the patient (client). Empowerment of the client/patient enhances the responsibility of the client for making decisions about his/her health. To impose a ban on the use of drugs in sport by competent adults would be considered an unwarranted intrusion into their lives and unjustified paternalism.

However, paternalism is not in itself an invalid basis for establishing an anti-doping policy, although the most common basis for paternaliism is the lack of competence of the other person due, for example, to coercion, ignorance or incapacity. In relation to adults, paternalism is often strongly resisted on the grounds that it conflicts with the principles associated with individual freedom dominant in western democracies.

Protecting athletes from themselves?

With regard to sport there are many individual sports which involve a substantial risk to the athlete's health and where, at first glance, paternalism might be supported. Even if one is reluctant to go as far as Fost does when he claims that "sport itself carries *per se* a substantial risk of death and permanent disability"[1], many would share the view of Lavin when he suggests that "Modern training regimens often keep players on the edge of injury".[2] Boxing is probably the clearest example of a sport where the risk to health is integral to the sport, but it can also be argued that there are many other sports where the probability of injury is great. Full contact sports such as American football, rugby union and rugby league can all provide examples of serious, and very occasionally, fatal injuries to participants. Mountaineering, and especially the current fashion for alpine-style climbing, has a long list of fatalities: for example, in May 1996, eleven climbers, using conventional mountaineering methods, lost their lives attempting to climb Everest. Even sports where the risk of fatal or serious injury is low, such as soccer and field hockey, pose a health risk to participants through repeated minor injury often resulting in chronic conditions such as arthritis. With the exception of the ban on boxing in a small number of countries and the recurring debate about its appropriateness in Olympic competition, there is little serious debate about banning high-risk sports.

A further weakness in relying on the desire to protect the health of the athlete as a justification for anti-doping policy is that there are many examples where athletes have competed with injuries without hindrance even when the risk of compounding the injury is substantial. The British runner Peter Elliot won a silver medal at the 1988 Olympics but was in such pain that he had to have five painkilling injections to enable him to run seven races in nine days. After the games, Elliot returned to Britain on crutches and needed a considerable period of physiotherapy before he was able to walk and run with ease. The use by athletes of analgesics and anti-inflammatory preparations is routine in almost all sports and, more importantly, the health of the athlete routinely comes second to the requirements of the team or squad. There seems little difference between the athletes who risk their health by competing when injured and the athletes who risk their health through the use of additive drugs.

If intervention to ban participation on health grounds fails with regard to sports where there is clear quantitative data on injury and fatalities, a similarly paternalistic rationale will not persuade with regard to drug use. As Fost notes "Even proving that an activity is harmful is therefore not a sufficient reason for preventing a competent person from pursuing that activity".[3] Consequently, even if the taking of anabolic steroids could be proved to be more dangerous than rugby, American football or mountaineering, the concern for the athlete's health would not provide a secure and plausible basis for supporting a ban on their use. Or put another way, if one is prepared to accept that concern for the athlete's health provides a sound basis for

---

1. Fost, N.C., op. cit., p. 481.
2. Lavin, M., op. cit., p. 37.
3. Fost, N.C., op. cit., p. 482.

intervention, then one would be obliged to pursue this logic and examine the many additional aspects of sports involvement which expose participants to health risks.

Approaching the issue from a different angle, Black and Pape provide a further challenge to anti-doping policy by arguing that the current attempts to impose a ban on drug use puts athletes' health at a greater risk than if the ban were lifted. They argue that reliance on the black market for drugs heightens the risk to the athlete because, *inter alia*, the purity of drugs cannot be guaranteed, advice about correct dosage is not available, and hygienic administration, especially of drugs taken intravenously, cannot be assured.[1] The conclusion drawn is that the ban on drug use is a greater threat to health than drug use itself. This argument has much in common with the case made against the policy of prohibition of alcohol in the United States. In other words the policy was more damaging than the problem it was seeking to solve.

A bad example to the young

A variation on this argument is that drug use, especially by elite athletes constantly in the public gaze, establishes harmful role models for children who may aspire to emulate not only the achievements of their heroes but also their methods. Unfortunately, this paternalistic rationale for banning doping is weakened by a number of inconsistencies. It is inconsistent because it is only considering one among many aspects of sport that might be considered dangerous. In order to be consistent it would be necessary to apply the same argument to the dangers arising from intensive training, training while injured, and potentially dangerous diets. The second source of inconsistency arises from the failure to apply the same argument, or at least to apply it so rigorously, to other potential role models for the young, especially from the music industry, television and cinema. The fact that many musicians, dancers and television and cinema stars have admitted to using drugs does not lead to a condemnation of their performance in the way that Ben Johnson's Olympic run was condemned. Third, the focus on the responsibility of elite athletes to set a good example to the young neglects the greater, or at least equal, burden of responsibility on the parents, coaches and teachers of the young. Unfortunately, comparing sportsmen and women with these other groups is of only limited value. Within music and the arts generally there is no strong view from either performers or audiences that these forms of entertainment should be drug-free, nor is there a situation where artists and performers publicly decry drug use while at the same time taking drugs in secret. There is clearly not the same sort of feeling among drug-free artists and the audience for the arts that drug abuse debases or devalues the spectacle or entertainment.

---

1. Black, T. & Pape, A. (1997), op. cit.

A stronger case can be made where the lack of experience of young people makes them especially vulnerable to misjudgements that might have long-term consequences for their health and wellbeing. Drug use would clearly come into this category where a decision based on information and experience cannot be expected from the young. The same argument can also be mounted when considering the capacity of young athletes to appreciate the risks in some training regimes. Young people are routinely subject to controls over their participation in sport that would not be applied to (or respected by) adults, such as non-swimmers wearing life preservers or identification wrist bands, or having to abide by different rules in "mini" versions of adult contact sports such as rugby.

Doping is the result of coercion

A further basis on which doping might be opposed is the claim that athletes do not take drugs freely but are coerced into drug use. At the heart of this argument is not the assumption that athletes are physically coerced to take drugs, but rather that athletes competing at the elite level are placed under intense peer or wider social pressure to take drugs. One version of this argument emphasises the narrowness of the gap between success and failure in many sports where the difference of less than 1% separates the winner from the athlete who comes in fourth or fifth. Athletes are consequently under intense pressure to take ever greater risks to find that extra centimetre or tenth (or hundredth) of a second: drug taking is simply one additional risk that they are compelled to take. As the sprinter, or more especially the high diver or gymnast, is being continually required to undertake increasingly intense training regimes or ever more complex and risky dives and routines so the pressure mounts on them to take that extra step and use drugs. Central to this argument is the assumption that drug use is rife at the elite level and that it is not possible to compete effectively at the top level unless one also takes drugs. In some ways this argument is also paternalistic, but intervention is justified on the basis of preventing the actions of one person (the drug user) causing harm to another (the non-drug user) rather than simply being justified on the basis of preventing injury or harm to oneself. The question that needs to be addressed is whether the harm to other, clean athletes, justifies the restrictions on the rights of the drug user.

The weaknesses of the argument based on coercion are clear. Unless one is referring to sport within repressive political regimes, athletes are always able to refuse drugs and simply to settle for fourth place or worse. Moreover, the reliance on an argument which justifies drug use on the grounds that "everyone at the top takes them" is untenable because of the lack of empirical evidence to sustain it, and also because the low ethical standards of others provides no justification for lowering one's own. In addition, the same argument is not heard in relation to other similar pressures. For example, if some athletes adopt a more intensive training regime which is perceived as successful, would a claim of coercion be made, let alone sustained, by the other athletes who emulated it? Drug use provides no greater basis for the claim of coercion than does particular dietary regimes, warm weather training, hypnosis or any other aspect of athletic preparation. If coercion is accepted as a possible basis for intervention, a further problem arises with regard to the difficulty of defining the point at which peer or social pressure becomes coercion.

A variation on this argument suggests that coercion arises from the inability of the athlete to provide informed consent to the use of drugs. It can be argued that modern elite athletes are surrounded by an array of experienced professional advisors, coaches, physiotherapists, doctors, dieticians, psychologists, etc., and are locked into an unequal relationship of professional and client. The disempowerment of athletes is best reflected by the way they are treated in many team sports as mere commodities to be traded between team owners with only minimal consultation and little regard for their interests. Athletes are, therefore, expected to fulfil a passive role within sport and the development of dependent relationships with professional staff is often encouraged. The weakness of this view is the profound difficulty in identifying the point at which the individual athlete cannot be held responsible for his or her actions. Even if athletes are locked into heavily dependent relationships, there has been so much publicity surrounding the anti-doping policy that it is hardly plausible for an athlete to deny knowledge of the policy and claim that they were unable to exercise their right to walk away from drug-based sport.

Even if one is prepared to entertain the argument that the source of coercion is not external to the athlete but an inner compulsion, the argument is still weak. To suggest that those who compete successfully at the highest levels display signs of psychological disturbance is not new. It is frequently suggested that elite athletes are obsessional and are simply not capable of making rational judgements about what is in their own best interests and will consequently takes risks with their health that "normal" people would not. However, even if this hypothesis were to be accepted, psychological imbalance might constitute a mitigating factor in defence of drug taking but it does not provide a justification for abuse.

A variation on this argument is that athletes in many sports are from poorer sections of society and from poorer countries and that they are under significant pressure because of the importance of sport as an escape route from poverty. Their social situation of vulnerability and marginalisation, so the argument runs, coerces them into making choices and taking risks that someone from a wealthier background is able to avoid. Poverty, as is the case with psychological disorder, might (and only might) provide a basis for mitigation but it does not provide a justification for doping. This is not simply because in some sports, boxing for example, the majority of competitors are from similarly poor backgrounds, but because individuals cannot be so easily freed from taking responsibility for their own actions and the desire to "get rich quick" is one of the least plausible.

Doping undermines the integrity of sport

The argument that doping conflicts with the core values of sport is strongly expressed by Schneider and Butcher who argue that "what is required is (..) a reaffirmation of the fundamental values of sport and the clarification of the mixed messages that the Olympic sports hierarchy currently sends out".[1] One presentation of this argument emphasises the extent to which sports are held as essentially related to games in that both are rule-governed activities and that games are defined in terms of their specific rules. If the rules of a particular game are broken then one cannot continue to claim that one is still playing that game. For example, if a soccer player picks up the ball and runs with it, he is no longer playing soccer. In the same way, if the rules prohibit drug use and a participant takes drugs then he or she has ceased to play that game and is playing a new game. This argument is attractive as it is more convincing to see anti-doping rules as being of a similar character to the rules that define the mode and form of play.

While each sport may claim, and may well have, an identifiable essence, all sports attempt to provide a mix of skills and challenges that make for a "good contest". Thus one might argue that for each sport it is possible to describe the particular mix of characteristics that the sport is designed to test. It might therefore be argued that one criterion for deciding whether doping should be banned is whether it undermines or invalidates the essential test or challenge of the sport. Gardner illustrates this argument by referring to the development and subsequent banning of u-grooved clubs in golf. It was claimed that u-groove clubs gave players better control over the flight of the ball especially out of the rough, with the poorer quality players gaining the greater advantage. The decision to outlaw the u-groove club was not because its use gave less talented golfers an advantage over the more talented but rather that it gave golfers in general an "advantage" over the sport itself, or at least an important element of it, namely the test of playing out of the rough: "what is being objected to here is not that performance enhancement will create inequality among athletes, but that it will lead to parity. In the end, u-grooves are more responsible for the performance than the golfer."[2] Extending this discussion, it has been suggested strongly in Formula One motor racing that the driver's contribution to success is increasingly marginal. When the Williams team decided not to renew Damon Hill's contract, despite the fact that he had just won the world championship, it was partly explained by the alleged view within the Williams' team camp that any

1. Schneider, A.J. & Butcher, R.B., "The Mesalliance of the Olympic Ideal and Doping, Why they Married and Why they Should Divorce", in Landry, F., Landry, M. & Yerles, M. (eds.), *Sport ... The Third Millennium*, Sainte-Foy, Les Presses de l' Université de Laval (1991), p. 495.
2. Gardner, R., op. cit. (1989), p. 69.

top class driver could win in a Williams car and that having the best driver was not a necessary condition. Sidestepping the question of whether Damon Hill is in fact the best Formula One driver in the world, it can be argued that, in general, the preferred relationship between the athlete and any equipment that he or she might use is one where a greater contribution to success is made by the former rather than the latter.

An extension of this argument is that sport encapsulates some deeper, more profound sense of humanity to which the rules of particular sports merely approximate and which drug use challenges and corrupts. Notwithstanding the difficulty of empirically verifying such an assertion, there is also the problem of responding to the equally attractive counter claim that sport, just like religion, is a social construction and imposes no prior obligation on the individual. A similar argument, voiced by Schneider and Butcher, is that drug use undermines the essential humanity of the athlete. According to this view, "one could describe the essence of sporting competition and excellence as the drive to perfect one aspect, the physical, of what it is to be human".[1] However, this attempt to identify the essence of humanity is as weak as the previous attempt to identify the essence of sport. As discussed above, the distinction between what is essential and what is not in sport is far from easy to draw.

Simon adopts a slightly different approach suggesting that "competition in athletics is best thought of as a mutual quest for excellence ... Competitors are obliged to do their best so as to bring out the best in their opponents".[2] For Simon the stress is on the mutual obligation of the athlete to maintain the essential aspect of sport as a competition between persons. The opponent is therefore not an obstacle to success, to be overcome by whatever means, but a co-worker in a joint undertaking. Simon's view is clearly at odds with the populist wisdom that winning is everything and postulates that the cliché, "taking part is more important than winning", is at best wistful nostalgia. Yet among sports enthusiasts there is likely to be a high level of agreement that, in track events for example, increasingly fast times are not the only criterion by which a good or enjoyable event is determined. The process by which the outcome is reached is also important: strategy, skill and stamina, for example, are some of the many ingredients of successful sport. Taking this view, "athletic competition, rather than being incompatible with respect for our opponents as persons, actually presupposes it".[3] Drug use tests merely how one body reacts to drugs by comparison to another. Any improvements in performance are due to how a person's body responds to the drug and does not reflect the person's hard work, dedication and skills and is not founded on respect for one's co-competitors. Simon acknowledges that his position rests

---

1. Ibid, p. 499 (emphasis in the original).
2. Simon, R.L. "Good Competition and Drug-Enhanced Performance", *Journal of the Philosophy of Sport*, Vol. XI, pp. 6-13 (1984), p. 10.
3. Ibid., p. 10.

on an ability to sustain the view that his conceptualisation of sport has a privileged moral standing. Indeed, Brown criticises Simon for basing his argument on a foundation that is "too vague to be persuasive".[1] Simon's position is further weakened by many of the criticisms of the attempts to distinguish between internal and external, and natural and unnatural advantages discussed in the earlier sections of this chapter. However, Simon's view is important in attempting to develop a plausible and persuasive normative rationale for an anti-doping policy and thus moving beyond the impasse arising from current attempts to secure a logically watertight foundation for policy.

Discussion

The preceding review has focused on a series of overlapping justifications for the current anti-doping policy. Justification has been sought in terms of the particular properties of drugs, a set of attributes associated with the athlete and a set of attributes associated with sport. Attempts to identify a set of morally objectionable qualities inherent in the current range of banned substances and practices is probably the weakest source of a viable policy rationale. There is no secure basis for objecting to advantages gained through using substances as it is only particular substances that are objected to and there are no definitive criteria that distinguish between the acceptable and the unacceptable. As Gardner notes there have been a number of attempts to distinguish "good" from "bad" substances such as distinguishing "food from non-food, restoratives from additives, [and] drugs from non-drugs", all with little success.[2]

Discussions that focus on the athlete and the effect of drugs on his/her natural state provide a stronger basis for the anti-doping policy but one which still has too many inconsistencies to provide a secure basis for policy. Much the same may be said of justifications based on claims regarding the particular properties of sport. However, it is this area, the nature of sport and the process by which it is socially constructed, that offers the most secure basis from which to defend current policy and to support its further refinement.

At first glance, the least satisfactory basis on which to justify banning drug use is that it is simply against the rules of particular sports. Rules are obviously imposed (and modified) for a purpose. That purpose might be to make a sport more exciting and attractive to spectators and television companies and viewers: rules might also be changed to make it more attractive to participants. Whatever the purpose might be, it undoubtedly has to be one that is understood by, and is persuasive to, participants, spectators and other interested parties. Consequently, if drug use is to be banned one must be able to answer the question "Why ban drug use?" in a convincing manner. For

---

1. Brown, W.M., "Comments on Simon and Fraleigh", *Journal of the Philosophy of Sport*, Vol. XI, pp. 33-35 (1985).
2. Gardner, R., op. cit. (1989), p. 66.

many supporters of the anti-doping policy, there appears to be a worryingly high number of opponents of the policy who argue cogently for its abandonment. The opponents of the anti-doping policy base their opposition on a mix of pragmatism and principle. The most commonly expressed pragmatic argument against current policy is to highlight the large number of inconsistencies and ambiguities in current policy. In addition, the opponents of the anti-doping policy argue that current policy implementation is inadequate and counterproductive as it creates greater inequality between the (covert) drug user and the non-user and that a more effective way of ensuring maximum fairness would be allow free use of drugs, on the assumption that any advantage would rapidly be competed away. Finally, there are those who oppose anti-doping efforts on the principled ground that it is an unwarranted interference with individual autonomy. In other words, not only is the current attempt to implement an anti-doping policy so flawed as to be doing more harm than good but also the extensive investment in the policy is based on a disregard for the fundamental rights of the individual. In Mill's classic statement of the liberal position, "the only purpose for which power can be rightfully exercised over any member of a civilised community, against his will, is to prevent harm to others. His own good, either physical or moral, is not a sufficient warrant.".[1] Not only does Mill provide a compelling argument for the sovereignty of the individual but it is a view that has been strongly in the ascendant over the last twenty years or so in much of the industrialised west and in Britain and the United States in particular.

Playing by the rules

It would appear that attempts to argue in favour of an anti-doping policy from "first principles" derived from the interests of the individual are difficult to sustain. If anti-doping policy is not rejected on the grounds that no rational person would introduce anti-doping rules if there is a chance that doping might compensate for some natural inequality, then it can be rejected on the grounds that the primary risks of drug use are borne by the taker and consequently do not constitute a sound basis for limiting the individual's rights to endanger themselves. Neither of these bases are without weaknesses that the supporter of doping control might exploit, but a more profitable avenue for reaching a publicly convincing basis for current policy is to abandon the search for an *a priori* rationale for policy and concentrate on middle order justifications which are derived from social experience. Such a shift of focus would bring the discussion back to the earlier theme of rules where it was suggested that doping should be rejected because it is a breach of the rules of the governing bodies of sport. In the earlier discussion, it was suggested that this was a weak foundation for anti-doping policy as it was based on a circular argument, namely that the use of anabolic steroids, for example, is

---

1. Mill, J.S., "On Liberty", in Warnock, M., *Utilitarianism, Essays of John Stuart Mill*, London, Fontana, p. 135.

cheating because their use is not allowed by the rules of sport. However, if we treat doping rules in the same way as we treat other rules of sport, that is as part of the agreement entered into by individuals before they are able to participate, then we are able to avoid the necessity or expectation that current rules have to be located in a set of principles that exist independent of the sport itself. There would not be any expectation that we should have to provide a rationale external to the sport of golf for the arbitrary rules that there shall be eighteen holes played rather than nineteen or that the ball shall be of a particular size. The rules depend for their survival on the extent to which they are able to command the respect and support of those who wish to play golf. This is not to argue that sport is an activity that is isolated from society and therefore does not need to take account of broader social opinion. Indeed, boxing has adjusted its rules on a number of occasions due to social concern at the risk of injury to participants.

At the heart of this position is the acceptance that sport is a socially constructed activity. The development of a satisfying sport that retains its popularity among both players and spectators is not the product of a rational calculation but rather the outcome of an often prolonged process of design, refinement and chance. The current rules and style of individual sports are the outcome of complex social processes which, while not unchanging, possess a considerable degree of inertia which gives them the permanence of social institutions. As such, sports reflect clusters of attitudes and values. The cluster of attitudes and values that describe and support a particular sport, and sport in general, are not limited to the rules and style of play but also cover contextual aspects of sport and include, *inter alia*, attitudes to the taking of particular drugs, the adoption of training regimes, and the financial rewards paid to athletes.

Lavin, in his examination of the ethics of drug use, proposes a similar way forward, but one which he admits is vulnerable to challenge. He suggests that even though there is widespread inconsistency among the general public and significant interest groups regarding doping, there is nonetheless a much higher level of consensus about which pharmaceutical preparations are considered acceptable and which are not and are subject to pervasive disapproval.[1] Pervasive disapproval is the product of a democratic process which far from claiming to encapsulate timeless values in sport is a product of a particular age, but which nonetheless captures the current core values of sport. Such a stance is consistent with the evidence available from the previous chapter where it was shown that the social perception of particular drugs, opium for example, is far from fixed and may move dramatically from tolerance and amusement to intolerance and demonisation.

---

1. Lavin, M., op. cit. p. 39.

The virtue of Lavin's position is that it accepts the absence of a tightly argued and philosophically watertight foundation for the prohibition on drug use, but also, and more importantly, acknowledges the need for a more pragmatic basis for current policy. Unless a more pragmatic response to the question "Why ban drug use?" can be established and defended, the inadequacies of attempts to build a rationale based on secure principle will continue to be exploited. Extending Lavin's position further one can argue that what is required is a popular and democratically secure basis for policy rather than an unassailable philosophical position. The various rationales for anti-doping policy that have been suggested above take the policy maker only so far along the road to policy implementation: it is the addition of the notion of democratic process that enables the completion of the journey. One would also hope that the tension between the rigour of philosophical argument and democratic decision would provide a degree of security that popular democracy will not lapse into mere populism, but also that the limitations of philosophical argument about drug use will not be too readily exploited by the unethical.

Balancing principle with popular support

The tension between philosophical principle and democratic opinion may be amply illustrated in current debates about many social issues including euthanasia, abortion and capital punishment. In all three of these areas of social policy, debates can be compartmentalised in terms of principle or opinion but in practice the philosophical debates inform, sensitise and respond to popular discussion. Policy positions based solely on principle are unsustainable unless there is popular support. In sport the clearest example of the problem of sustaining a policy based on principle without popular support is the gradual undermining of both amateurism and the exclusion of women from many sports during the twentieth century.

The search for a rationale for anti-doping policy within a democratic process is highly consistent with the current debates on communitarianism and the communitarian critique of liberal individualism. Communitarianism rejects liberal individualism in preference for a theory which argues that the self and aspects of social reality, including sporting values, relations, culture and institutions, are the products of social construction. Communitarianism has much in common with contemporary pragmatic philosophy which stresses the importance of seeking justifications for what we do in our daily practices rather than in the search for objective truths about the world. The dual strands in communitarian thought have substantial significance for the current debate on drugs in sport. The first strand is that it is not possible to conceive of the individual except as a member of his/her community and its practices and values. As Frazer and Lacey argue "the community constitutes the person. Social processes and institutions, the family, churches, political and educational systems, shape the infant into a social being who experiences emotion, who desires, who has understanding of and attitudes towards the social world and her place in it".[1] The implication of this view is clear for any discussion of the rules that should govern participation in sport and drug use in particular, namely that it is only possible to discuss the rights of the individual athlete to take drugs from within an understanding of the social institution of sport, that is as part of the web of human relationships that exist within sport in general and sporting competition in particular. The second strand of communitarianism concerns the development and "owner-ship" of values. The communitarian argument is that values are the product of, and are validated by, particular communities and do not proceed natural-ly from universal human nature as is commonly argued by the liberal individ-ualist. The assumption that human beings are essentially social results in an emphasis on those values that reinforce attitudes, beliefs and practices that acknowledge and reaffirm the communal and mutually supportive elements of human life. "Thus, reciprocity, solidarity, fraternity and community take the place of the liberal priorities such as fulfilment of individual rights and respect for individual freedom in the sphere of political value".[2]

The applicability of these views to the sporting community are obvious and provide a powerful rationale for the current anti-doping policy. The current anti-doping policy is seen as the product of the dominant values and atti-tudes within the contemporary sport community rather than the product of abstract principle. Consequently, the ambiguities and inconsistencies in cur-rent policy are not necessarily weaknesses in the policy but are rather reflec-tions of the differentiation between particular practices and substances that emerge from community experience and which reflect collective opinion. The attraction of the communitarian approach to policy justification is that it clearly roots the legitimacy of a policy in the level of popular support it com-mands. From the policy maker's point of view, an important aspect of suc-cessful policy implementation is the maintenance of the high level of support for the "pervasive disapproval" on which the credibility of the policy depends.

The dangers of basing anti-doping policy, or indeed any policy, solely on its capacity to generate support within a community are obvious. The confi-dence shown by communitarians in the common sense of democracy needs to be tempered with a reminder of how easily democratic common sense can slip towards arbitrary populism. In addition, the proponents of anti-doping would be in great difficulty if they were faced by a sports community which endorsed doping for they would have no basis on which to challenge the democratic will. Despite the attractions of communitarianism, the dangers of moral relativism are all too apparent. It is therefore important not to abandon

---

1. Frazer, E. & Lacey, N., *The Politics of Community: A Feminist Critique of the Liberal-Communitarian Debate*, Hemel Hempstead: Harvester-Wheatsheaf (1993), p. 108.
2. Ibid., pp.10-11.

the debate based on the more abstract notions of individual rights, fairness, harm and essence of sport as they might well be needed to provide constraints on the exercise of popular judgement. Indeed, among communitarians there are those such as Charles Taylor who moderate their defence of moral relativism by arguing strongly that community-derived values must be compatible with a set of deeper moral intuitions about the worth and dignity of other human beings, about what constitutes a good life and about what makes us worthy of the respect of others.

In conclusion, the quest for a set of universal and unassailable principles on which to base an anti-doping policy in sport is not capable of being fulfilled, although reference to the intuitive values that Taylor refers to gives some external justification for policies designed to eradicate doping. Current policy is, though, capable of being strongly defended on the basis of the weight of democratic community condemnation and pervasive disapproval. In many respects this is no different from the way that policy towards many other contemporary moral issues, abortion, divorce, treatment of prisoners in war, and treatment of refugees, is determined. Of over-riding importance is the fact that policy is consequently never secure but always in need of defence, support and refinement. The challenge to the sports authorities is to develop a persuasive definition of doping and a programme of policy implementation that takes account of the need to sustain popular disapproval of doping. Without strong community support for anti-doping the policy may suffer the same fate as other principled positions, such as that regarding amateurism, which gradually became unsustainable due to the erosion of public support and confidence.

Chapter 6

The evolution of anti-doping policy: problems and solutions

In any discussion of the current anti-doping policy it is important to bear in mind constantly just how recently the issue of doping in sport has been defined as a problem and how recently drug testing and other policy solutions have been introduced. Forty years ago there was not only no testing but little discussion of drug abuse within sport, apart from a small group of administrators, coaches and doctors. Thirty years ago the first tentative steps were taken towards developing a definition of doping and beginning the process of policy formulation. Twenty-five years ago there was only limited testing at major international and some national sports events. Twenty years ago the first steps were being taken to introduce out-of-competition testing. Given the recent history of anti-doping policy, it is hardly surprising that the pace of policy development has not slowed over recent years and that sports administrators argue that anti-doping policy is still characterised by its dynamism rather than its stability.

Tracing the evolution of policy involves examining the decisions of a number of different types of organisations. There are the sports bodies, the most significant of which is the International Olympic Committee. Other key sports organisations include a number of national sports confederations and the major international federations, particularly the International Amateur Athletic Federation. Paralleling the activities of these sports bodies are a number of government organisations. A leading role in debates on doping policy has consistently been taken by the Council of Europe with bodies such as the European Union and Unesco making occasional, but largely rhetorical, interventions. Finally, account must also be taken of the contribution of a number of individual governments to the shaping of policy in the early years of debate.

The evolution of anti-doping policy can also be traced along, at least, four main strands, namely clarification of policy focus, generation and maintenance of political commitment, technology development, and the establishment of the necessary resource infrastructure. Clarification of the focus refers to the progressive refinement of the broad categories and particular examples of drugs and doping practices targeted by the policy makers. The second dimension concerns the stimulation of political support for policy implementation. Here the focus is not just on governments and sports authorities but also on athletes and the general public and is a continuing activity. Not only is the progressive widening and deepening of the coalition of support a benefit to the supporters of the anti-doping policy, it is also a requirement for the continuance of policy momentum that each significant policy development stimulates a round of routine maintenance and reinforcement of that coalition of support. The third dimension refers to technological demands; effective policy implementation depends substantially on the development of testing and analytical techniques and their continuing refinement to match the advances in pharmacology and the deviousness of drug-abusing athletes. The final dimension directs attention to the resource infrastructure which supports policy implementation and includes the provision of money, laboratories, sampling officers and a regulatory framework.

Until the mid 1960s, concern about doping had been limited to a relatively small group of specialists within sport and the private concern had not yet become a public issue. The series of high profile scandals in the early to mid 1960s forced the issue on to the agenda of both governments and sports bodies. A series of doping incidents in the previous years and especially the death of the Danish cyclist, Kurt Jensen, at the 1960 Rome Olympics prompted a convention in January 1963 of European sports governing bodies. One outcome of this meeting was the provision of a definition of doping which was later adopted by the International Olympic Committee and the International Doping Conference of the Fédération Internationale de Medecine Sportive in Tokyo in 1964. Doping was defined as "the administration to, or the use by, a competing athlete of any substance foreign to the body or any physiological substance taken in abnormal quantity or by an abnormal route of entry into the body, with the sole intention of increasing in an artificial and unfair manner his performance in competition".[1]

The weaknesses of this early definition are obvious. The difficulty with phrases such as "any substance foreign to the body", substances taken in "abnormal quantities", "abnormal route of entry", or "with the sole intention ..." are too obvious to require further elaboration. This early attempt at specifying the problem to be tackled marked the start of a period of intense discussion by all the key bodies interested in the definition of doping. Incidents of doping associated with cycling were again the stimulus to action, this time by the Council of Europe rather than the federations. The refusal by the five leading cyclists taking part in the 1966 world road race championships to provide a urine sample, and the death a year later of a professional rider in the Tour de France, caused substantial public criticism and discussion and prompted the Council of Europe to debate and pass a resolution condemning doping by athletes.

The condemnation was justified on grounds of health, poor example to the young and that doping was contrary to the spirit of fair play in sport. Included in the resolution was a definition of doping as the "administration to or use by a healthy person, in any manner whatsoever, of agents foreign to the

---

1. Barnes, L. "Olympic Drug Testing, Improvement without Progress", *Physician and Sports Medicine*, Vol. 8, (1980).

organism, or of physiological substances in excessive quantities or introduced by an abnormal channel, with the sole purpose of affecting artificially and by unfair means the performance of such a person when taking part in a competition".[1] This definition attempts to resolve some of the ambiguities of the 1964 definition, but the additional phrases (such as the reference to the use of drugs by "a healthy person") compounded the problems and consequently shared many of the weaknesses of the 1964 attempt. Despite the continuing problems in arriving at an operational definition, the Council resolution also included a recommendation to its member governments to encourage their sports associations and federations to initiate action to condemn doping and to penalise offenders. Probably the most important statement within the resolution was the exhortation to member states to encourage their federations to apply anti-doping regulations "to any person who, in another member state, has been penalised".[2] The significance of the statement lay in its recognition of the international nature of the emerging problem and foreshadowed the current emphasis on harmonisation of policy between federations and between countries.

Drug testing

While the political momentum was growing for a policy to challenge doping, the deficiencies of current technology were becoming all too apparent. In the 1960s, the early tests were focused on cycling and were directed at the detection of amphetamines, the most widely used drug. Although there was an awareness of the increasing use of anabolic steroids, there was no reliable test for this class of drugs. As regards testing for amphetamines, "early testing methods were relatively unsophisticated: the technology available to analyse an athlete's urine resulted in inaccurate findings that failed to deter drug use".[3]

The intervention by the Council of Europe in the 1960s was significant, not only because it responded to a wave of public concern about the issue of doping in sport but also because it was a sharp reminder to international sports organisations that governments also had an interest in the issue. Paralleling the growing interest of the Council of Europe an increasing number of individual governments were introducing legislation or regulations aimed at drug abuse in sport. As early as 1965, the governments of France and Belgium legislated against doping, followed by Turkey and Italy in 1971. Consequently, the action by the Council and the increasing threat of legislation by individual governments spurred the IOC and a number of key international federations, such as the Union Cycliste Internationale and the IAAF into action. The IOC had for many years been wary of government interest

---

1. Council of Europe Resolution (67) 12 on the doping of athletes, adopted 20 June 1967.
2. Ibid., paragraph 1.c.
3. Verroken, M. & Mottram, D.R. "Doping Control in Sport", in Mottram, D.R. (ed.), *Drugs in Sport*, London, E & FN Spon (1996), p. 235.

and involvement in sport and particularly Olympic sport.[1] Although the IOC had established a Medical Commission in 1961 and passed a resolution condemning doping as early as 1962, it was not until five years later that it re-established and re-invigorated the Medical Commission so that it should advise the IOC and oversee the development of policy. Limited testing was introduced by international federations in mid to late 1960s, with FIFA being among the first when it announced that tests would be carried out at the 1966 Soccer World Cup in England. Two years later tests were conducted at the winter and summer Olympic Games in Grenoble and Mexico City respectively, followed by testing at the 1970 Commonwealth Games and the 1974 European Athletics Championships. In these early years very few positive results were recorded, not only because there was an uncertainty about the reliability of the tests, but more importantly because there was a marked lack of clarity about where the primary responsibility for the implementation of testing lay. As is so often the case with new policy initiatives, initial enthusiasm was slowly being replaced with a growing appreciation of the organisational and financial costs of effective testing. This was particularly true for event-organising bodies, such as the IOC and the Commonwealth Games Federation and for the international federations, none of whom were financially strong. Even the IOC was at that time a relatively modest body relying substantially on voluntary activity and the largesse of host countries.

The IOC, for example, clearly saw its responsibility limited to alerting national Olympic committees to the need to promote drug-free sport and to ensure that local organising committees for Olympic Games made arrangements for testing. It made a point of stating that the organising of testing is "a responsibility that the International Olympic Committee is not prepared to take".[2] Despite the obvious reluctance by the IOC to adopt a central policy role it has steadily increased its involvement in the policy area, most notably through the accreditation of laboratories for the analysis of samples and also through the maintenance of what has become the benchmark list of banned substances and practices, producing the first such list in 1971. Where the IOC has drawn the line is at extending its involvement in the administration of testing beyond IOC-sanctioned competitions.

The first Olympic Games at which there was reasonably comprehensive testing across all events was the 1972 Munich Games when just over 2000 tests were conducted and seven athletes disqualified. Tests were conducted for narcotic analgesics and for stimulants, but not for anabolic steroids as no reliable tests had yet been developed and the IOC was unwilling to list a substance for which there was no test. By the mid 1970s testing for stimulants was sufficiently accurate to provide a deterrent against the use of the most

---

1. See Houlihan, B., *Sport and International Politics*, Hemel Hempstead, Harvester-Wheatsheaf (1994) for a discussion of the tensions in the relationship between the Olympic movement and international government bodies such as Unesco, the EU and the Council of Europe.
2. IOC Newsletter, August 1968, quoted in Verroken & Mottram, op. cit. p. 236.

common drugs in this class, such as amphetamines. However, by the early 1970s it was acknowledged that the major drugs abused by athletes were no longer stimulants but steroids. Whereas tests for amphetamines and most other stimulants were easy and cheap to devise as they merely required the adaptation of existing analytical procedures, the development of a test for steroids required original research which had to be funded. The breakthrough came early in the 1970s when a reliable test for many drugs in the steroid class was developed by Professor Raymond Brooks. The radioimmunoassay test was piloted at the 1972 Olympic Games under the direction of Dr Manfred Donike and was officially used at the 1976 Montreal Games with the drug having been added to the IOC list the previous year. Eight athletes were disqualified from the games due to positive test results for steroids. Over the next ten years the IOC gradually expanded its list of banned substances and practices through the addition of testosterone and caffeine in the early 1980s, beta-blockers and blood-doping in 1985, and diuretics in 1987 (see Table 6.1).

Table 6.1: Substances identified by IOC-accredited laboratories 1986-96

Substance	1986	1987	1988	1989	1990	1991	1992	1993	1994	1995	1996
Anabolic steroids	439	521	791	611	579	652	717	995	891	986	1131
Stimulants	177	301	420	508	340	221	277	339	347	310	281
Narcotics	23	55	58	76	62	72	102	48	42	34	37
Beta-blockers	31	33	8	6	8	10	12	13	15	14	6
Diuretics	2	9	57	45	37	47	70	66	63	59	54
Masking agents	*	24	19	10	6	1	22	23	8	3	0
Peptide hormones	*	*	*	*	1	1	4	4	3	9	4
Total	672	943	1353	1256	1033	1004	1204	1488	1369	1415	1513

* not tested
Source: IOC statistics

While the IOC was reluctant to adopt a leading role in global policy development, it was forced to become more deeply involved in a number of aspects of anti-doping policy implementation, if for no other reason than to protect the integrity of the Olympic Games. The accreditation of laboratories is one such example. Some work on accrediting laboratories had been undertaken by the IAAF in the mid 1970s which did much to inform the protocols adopted by the IOC in 1976 for initial accreditation and in 1985 for re-accreditation. Accreditation was introduced primarily in an attempt to protect the IOC and international federations from legal challenge to the procedures adopted within laboratories. Currently accredited laboratories are subject to re-accreditation on an annual basis and have their analytical standards tested every four months. The work undertaken by the IOC in establishing quality standards for laboratories dealing with urine samples from Olympic Games has resulted in the IOC requirements becoming the *de facto* standards for all

133

sports drug analysis laboratories such that many non-Olympic sports send their samples to IOC-accredited laboratories. Although the IOC deserves much credit for developing quality standards for laboratories, there is still some concern that there is no independent verification that laboratories have met the IOC standards or deserved re-accreditation. Justice Dubin during his inquiry into drug use by athletes in Canada considered that the practice of members of the IOC subcommission who granted accreditation also being heads of IOC-accredited laboratories constituted a conflict of interest.

Many of those closely involved in shaping IOC policy on doping were also involved in similar discussions within their own international federations. Not surprisingly, given the centrality of track and field events to the Olympics, the IAAF was particularly closely involved in IOC deliberations, with its policy making keeping in close step with that of the IOC. The IAAF formed its Medical Committee in 1972 and placed both blood doping and anabolic steroids on its list of banned practices and substances even though reliable tests were not yet firmly in place. In 1976 the federation formed a doping sub-commission and a year later introduced mandatory doping control at federation championships. Progress towards agreeing a set of penalties for breaches of doping regulations was slower, but by 1978 the federation had introduced a minimum suspension of eighteen months for doping infractions. Eight years later the federation began a process of refinement of penalties when it modified its policy to differentiate between unintentional use (for example of ephedrine which is a common ingredient in many over-the-counter medicines) for which the penalty was to be a suspension of three months for a first offence, and a set of stronger penalties for the use of major drugs such as steroids where the penalty was to be a ban of two years for a first offence. A second offence concerning ephedrine or its derivatives resulted in a ban of two years with a life ban for a third offence. A life ban was to be imposed for a second offence concerning a major drug.

Gathering momentum

The late 1980s marked the start of a period of intense policy development. In 1987 the IAAF supported the first in a series of symposia on doping organised under the aegis of the International Athletic Foundation and aimed at raising the profile of the issue among athletes and also providing a forum for discussing aspects of implementation. The Göteborg Manifesto, accepted by the IAAF in 1989, was supported by an extensive series of changes in policy including the establishment of a "flying squad" of sampling officers, the arrangement for world-recognised visas for flying squad members to prevent countries taking advantage of advance warning of their arrival, and the provision of financial support to domestic governing bodies to support testing programmes.

By the 1970s the Council of Europe was beginning to treat doping as an aspect of a broader policy relating to the maintenance of ethical standards within sport. Consequently, references to doping were made within the context of related policy statements such as that on "Sport for All" in 1976. Within the European Sport for All Charter, itself a series of moral imperatives, Article V provides the exhortation that "methods shall be sought to safeguard sport and sportsmen from exploitation for political, commercial or financial gain, and from practices that are abusive and debasing, including the unfair use of drugs". This position was reinforced at the 2nd Conference of European Ministers responsible for Sport held in 1978 at which Prince Alexandre de Merode, President of the IOC Medical Commission, reported on the substantial problems in making progress in encouraging domestic sports organisations and international federations to adopt rigorous anti-doping measures.[1] The second conference adopted a resolution which again linked opposition to doping to a strong statement on the ethics of sport, but went further than the earlier statement by identifying the main agents of policy implementation and the steps that should be taken in developing an effective policy response to the problem. Although the statement was directed towards member governments, it was acknowledged that policy formulation and especially implementation would require the support and resources of domestic and international sports bodies. However, it was recognised that governments had an important role to play in the provision of specialist facilities to support drug testing, such as analytic laboratories, and also in facilitating the development of an internationally co-ordinated response. More importantly, the conference identified a series of key aspects of successful policy development, many of which remain issues of continuing concern. The first aspect concerned the need to compile and publish an "accurate and detailed lists of stimulating agents and means of testing for them" ; the second referred to the need to identify ways of "instituting and supporting practical and regular doping tests" both "at and between events" ; while the third concerned "instituting stricter sanctions for athletes found using stimulants, which should also be applied to trainers, doctors or managers who have encouraged their use" supported by a "publicity campaign directed at athletes on the dangers to health of doping". These three issues, agreeing the list of proscribed practices and substance, the testing process, and the penalties to be applied and to whom, are recurring themes in the refinement of anti-doping policy.

During the late 1970s and early 1980s, the lead on debating and developing policy on anti-doping policy lay, publicly at least, with the IOC and increasingly with the IAAF. However, it should be borne in mind that the Council of Europe and a number of individual governments played a significant part in encouraging the Olympic movement to adopt a policy leadership role. The

---

1. By the early 1970s action was being taken by a number of national sports organisations including the Deutscher Sportbund of the Federal Republic of Germany and the Norwegian Confederation of Sport, generally taking their lead from the IOC, but in the case of the Norwegian Confederation providing a lead to other federations and to the IOC.

IOC's centrality to policy making on doping was in part through intent and partly through a concern not to lose, by default, control over a high profile issue in sport to governments. In reality, policy making on doping was rapidly emerging as inherently a twin-track process where the relationship between sports organisations, on the one hand, and governments and international governmental bodies, on the other, hovered between mutual support and reinforcement of common objectives and mutual suspicion that the other was either subverting the policy or was attempting to dominate the policy arena.

Scientific advances: keeping ahead of the drug abuser?

Paralleling developments in the political relationship between sporting and government organisations was the steady progress in the refinement of sample analysis techniques. Although the breakthrough in the development of a test for anabolic steroids in the mid 1970s resulted in the apprehension of a number of drug abusers, it did little to stem the rapid increase in the popularity of the drug. While radioimmunoassay was successful in identifying the presence of a number of steroids, it was less successful with the more sophisticated drugs in the class and also less successful in identifying very small traces of the drug. As Robert Voy, one-time chief medical officer of the United States Olympic Committee, notes, "before 1983 drug testing and detection at all international competitions was very ineffective, simply because the technology was primitive and undependable".[1] Pre-1983 testing produced not only false negatives but also false positives with the result that athletes were often able to appeal against decisions on the grounds that the outcome of the test could not be guaranteed beyond reasonable doubt. Voy also pointed to the inadequacies of sampling procedures, especially the inability of doping agencies to guarantee the security of the "chain of custody" and therefore to state authoritatively that tampering or contamination of the sample could not have occurred. The deficiencies in the collection process provided "the biggest opportunity to challenge the testing system".[2] The main consequence of the weaknesses in procedures and the fear of legal challenge was that sports authorities would only proceed with the small number of test results that were deemed to be unchallengeable and many positive results were ignored. By the early 1980s, new and more sensitive detection methods were available based on gas chromatography/mass spectrometry (GC/MS) which was capable of identifying traces of steroids as small as one part per billion. In addition to enabling testing for anabolic steroids, GC/MS was also able to indicate the level of testosterone in the athletes' urine. It was the announcement that GC/MS analysis was to be used on samples from the 1983 Pan-American Games that led to the high number

---

1. Voy, R., *Drugs, Sport and Politics, The Inside Story About Drug Use in Sport and its Political Cover-up*, Champaign, Ill., Leisure Press, p. 77.
2. Ibid., p. 78.

of withdrawals by athletes prior to the games and the high number of positives at the games. The increasing use of anabolic steroids that gave such urgency to the search for analytic methods and technology to enable their detection also led anti-doping authorities to a realisation that the deterrence value of effective competition testing was undermined by the use of steroids as training aids rather than competition aids. More importantly, it was also realised that the introduction of GC/MS technology was being used by unscrupulous athletes to determine the excretion time for different drugs in order to identify when they needed to stop taking the drug prior to competition.

The mid to late 1970s was the period when the move to introduce out-of-competition testing was made, not with the intention of replacing in-competition testing, but rather to complement it. Norway was one of the first countries to introduce out-of-competition testing. Its initial programme was introduced in 1977 with the proportion of total tests conducted out-of-competition rising to over 70% by the late 1980s. Britain was typical of the majority of countries that began to introduce out-of-competition testing during the mid 1980s. In Britain, this form of testing was introduced by the British Amateur Athletic Board on a pilot basis with Sports Council funding in 1985. In 1988 the practice was adopted by a broader group of governing bodies due, in large part, to encouragement and financial support from the Sports Council. One of the most significant lessons learnt from the early experience of out-of-competition testing was the need to develop a procedure that was adapted to the increasingly international training and competition schedules of elite athletes. If short notice, or preferably no-notice, testing was to be effective, it was essential that governing bodies knew where athletes were throughout the year. There were too many instances of athletes deliberately selecting inaccessible locations for training or "forgetting" to inform their governing body of their movements. The process of establishing a testing infrastructure appropriate to an increasingly internationalised athletic community has been slow and is not yet complete. However, there have been some moves to develop the necessary framework for implementation. In 1988, GAISF gave its support to out-of-competition testing as did the European Sports Conference a year later. Of especial importance was the decision, in 1989, by the IAAF council to impose random testing on all international-level athletes thus by-passing any domestic governing bodies that had been dragging their feet on the issue. In May 1990, the first IAAF "flying squad" of testing officers visited the then Soviet Union, followed by visits to France and Italy.

The role of the Council of Europe

For the Council of Europe the next notable stage in its contribution to the policy process was the formulation of a recommendation to member governments prompted by the 1978 Ministers Conference. The recommendation left aside the increasingly difficult question of the definition of doping and concentrated on the more practical issues of implementation. In the recommendation the emerging issue was that of harmonisation of policy between federations. There was also some elaboration of earlier policy tools. For example, the earlier emphasis on the need to publicise to athletes the dangers of drug use was expanded to include coaches and administrators. Emphasis was also placed on the need for investment in the scientific resources, especially laboratories, necessary to support an effective testing regime. At the time of formulating the recommendation, there were only three IOC-approved laboratories in the twenty-two member states of the Council of Europe.

The work of the Council was paralleled within the Olympic movement. Of particular importance was the 11th Olympic Congress in Baden-Baden in 1981 where a resolution from athletes gave legitimacy and added momentum to the IOC's anti-doping activity. The Baden-Baden appeal also added to the growing interest within the Council and its advisory groups in developing a comprehensive policy statement in the form of an Anti-doping Charter. The significance of the Anti-Doping Charter was primarily as a public statement of commitment by governments to the anti-doping campaign. The charter was also of value as a benchmark and focus for policy development at the national level and as an important symbol of the elimination of doping as a joint endeavour by sports and governmental organisations. The text of the charter was drafted by an expert committee chaired by Prince Alexandre de Merode who played, and continues to play, a central role in the IOC's anti-doping efforts.

The charter was adopted in 1984 and was, at one level, an expression of political intent to tackle the issue of doping.[1] However, at a more significant level, it provided a series of recommendations for the construction of an effective policy response to doping at the domestic and at the international levels in terms of the provision of resources to support the efforts of sports organisations to counter doping. Legislation was suggested to restrict the availability of drugs likely to be used in sport doping and financial support was recommended to help meet the cost of testing. Member governments were also encouraged to facilitate the harmonisation of anti-doping regulations and procedures among governing bodies using the IOC and IAAF recommended regulations and procedures as a guide. The status of the charter was that of a recommendation, though it was hoped that "it would have a moral, political and practical impact higher than that of an ordinary recommendation".[2] Although it is always wise to be wary of ascribing too much significance to public expressions of support for statements of intent, the charter did generate considerable interest among both government and

---

1. A copy of the charter is included in *The Council of Europe's Work on Sport 1967-91*, Vol. 1, Strasbourg, Council of Europe (1992), pp. 63-66.
2. Council of Europe "Explanatory Report on the Anti-Doping Convention", Strasbourg, Council of Europe (1990).

non-government organisations. Within twelve months of publication, the General Association of International Sports Federations and the IOC had both passed resolutions endorsing the charter and in 1985 the Association of European National Olympic Committees also expressed its support. Acknowledgements of the status of the charter came from Unesco, the European Community and the World Health Organisation. At around the same time, countries outside Europe were also showing interest in using the charter as the basis for shaping domestic policy, with Canada being an early supporter. In late 1987, and with more than a trace of irony, a group of sports organisations in socialist states contacted the Council of Europe with a request for a set of internationally accepted rules and obligations on doping. The following year, in June 1988, the 1st Permanent World Conference on Anti-Doping was held in Ottawa and co-chaired by the IOC and Canada. Of particular importance was the adoption by the conference of an International Doping Charter, later endorsed by the IOC and retitled the Olympic Anti-Doping Charter, modelled very closely on the Council of Europe charter.

By the late 1980s, the issue of doping had moved from being a marginal subject in sport with discussion limited to a core of experts and "insiders" to being an issue which held centre-stage in a series of sporting and non-sporting organisations and also increasingly within the media. In addition, although in public the relationship between governmental and non-governmental bodies was one of mutual support, it disguised an underlying tension. The basis of unease among governments and government organisations was not so much an explicit distrust of the commitment of either the IOC or the major federations to anti-doping but rather a more general concern with their reliance on self-regulation in preference to inviting an independent agency to take responsibility for anti-doping policy implementation. On the other hand, sports organisations were suspicious of the motives of governments, particularly at a time when the prestige and public relations opportunities afforded by Olympic Games and other major international sports events were becoming increasingly apparent.

The decision of the Council of Europe to redesignate the charter as a convention which member states would be asked to sign and which non-member states would be invited to support was a mark of the progress that had been made over the previous ten years in raising the profile of the issue and was also a recognition that co-ordination at the international level by both sporting and non-sporting bodies was essential for effective implementation (see Appendix B for the text of the convention). The focus of the convention was on harmonisation of policy between countries and between sports. As in the charter, the emphasis in the convention was on policy implementation through sports organisations although it was clearly acknowledged that the resources of the state, whether legislative or financial, were essential for successful implementation. The early concern to provide a comprehensive definition of doping was replaced by a less problematic statement that "doping in sport" means the administration to sportsmen or sportswomen, or the use by them, of pharmacological classes of doping agents or doping methods".[1] Pharmacological classes of doping agents or doping methods were simply defined as those "classes of doping agents or doping methods banned by the relevant international sports organisation".[2]

The preparation of the convention marked a watershed in the activity of the Council on anti-doping policy not just because there was a now a benchmark against which to measure the commitment of other countries but also because it coincided with the collapse of the governments and sporting infra-structures in the communist countries of central and eastern Europe. The need in these countries to rebuild sports organisations with often negligible state support was an opportunity for the Council to provide advice and sup-port, not only on sports infrastructure but also on the importance of re-affirming a set of sports values that incorporated a strong anti-doping ele-ment. Indeed, as Table 6.2 shows, for many ex-communist countries accession to both the European Cultural Convention and the Anti-doping Convention was a common precursor to an invitation from the Council of Ministers to join the Council of Europe itself.

Table 6.2: Incorporation of countries of central and eastern Europe into the Council of Europe (in chronological order)

Country	Accession to ECC[1]	Accession to ADC[1]	Membership of CE[1]
Hungary	Nov. 1989	Jan. 1990	Nov. 1990
Poland	Nov. 1989	June 1990	Nov. 1991
Czech Republic	May 1990*	April 1995	June 1993
Slovakia	May 1990*	May 1993	June 1993
Russian Federation**	Feb. 1991**	Feb. 1991**	Feb. 1996
Bulgaria	Sep. 1991	June 1992	May 1992
Romania	Dec. 1991	Dec. 1998	Oct. 1993
Estonia	May 1992	Nov. 1997	May 1993
Latvia	May 1992	Jan. 1997	Feb. 1995
Lithuania	May 1992	May 1996	May 1993
Albania	June 1992		July 1995
Slovenia	July 1992	July 1992	May 1993
Croatia	Jan. 1993	Jan. 1993	Nov.1996
Belarus	Oct. 1993		
Moldova	May 1994	July 1995	
Ukraine	June 1994	Nov.1995	
Bosnia and Herzegovina	Dec. 1994	Dec. 1994	
"The former Yugoslav Republic of Macedonia"	Nov.1995	Mar..1994	Nov.1995
Armenia	April 1997		
Azerbaijan	April 1997		
Georgia	April 1997		

Notes:
* when Czechoslovakia
** when the former Soviet Union
1. ECC (European Cultural Convention); ADC (Anti-doping Convention); CE (Council of Europe)
Source: Council of Europe

---

1. Council of Europe Anti-doping Convention (1989) Article 2, Paragraph 1, section a.
2. Ibid., Article 2, paragraph 1, section b.

The late 1980s: scandal and policy review

The late 1980s marked a watershed in policy development not just for the ex-communist countries but also for some of the countries that had considered themselves to be occupying the moral high ground on the issue of doping. In Australia, the United Kingdom and Canada, scandal, allegations of abuse and suspicion of collusion by sporting authorities in covering up positive results raised the public and political profile of drugs in sport. For many Australians sporting success epitomised the character and qualities of the country, giving sport a particular prominence in Australian culture.[1] Sustained international sporting success in the post-war years was complemented by innovations in sports development activity which were frequently seen as models in the non-communist world of the 1980s. The publication of allegations of systematic drug abuse at the flagship elite sports development centre, the Australian Institute of Sport (AIS), in 1987, caused such a public outcry that a Senate Committee of Inquiry was established. At the heart of the allegations was the suggestion that coaches and administrators at the AIS had colluded with athletes to circumvent doping control procedures. The picture painted of Australian anti-doping policy was one of minimal compliance, and a culture which sought to test the boundaries of current policy. There was little harmonisation of policy among governing bodies and even less enthusiasm to give the issue priority over maximising the medal count at international sports competitions. Anti-doping policy in the mid 1980s, such as it was, was unco-ordinated and unenthusiastically implemented. Although over 500 athletes were covered by the testing programme it was, in the words of the athletics coach at the AIS, "regarded as a joke by athletes. In the case of track and field the only tested meet is usually the national championships and they know when that is on, so athletes can easily organise their schedules to avoid the testing".[2]

The inquiry highlighted a range of specific problems that included the lack of commitment from many athletes and coaches, the lack of confidence in the laboratories that undertook sample analysis, and the general unwillingness of governing bodies to provide a strong lead on anti-doping. In many respects these problems with effective policy implementation highlight the problems faced by anti-doping advocates arising from the context of modern sport. The lack of enthusiasm among athletes and coaches, especially those based at the AIS was, in part, a fear that they might lose the financial support that government gives to individual athletes if the level of achievement declined. Staff at the AIS were under considerable pressure to justify public expenditure on the facility through continued success in international competition.

---

1. For a more detailed discussion and analysis of the events at the AIS see Houlihan, B., *Sport, Policy and Politics, A Comparative Analysis*, London, Routledge (1997).
2. Australia, "Drugs in Sport", An Interim Report of the Senate Standing Committee on Environment, Recreation and the Arts (The Black Report), Canberra, Commonwealth of Australia (1989) p. 84.

Similarly there was a disincentive for governing bodies to pursue rigorously drug abusers as they too were dependent on Olympic success for the continuation of their government funding. This link between Olympic and international achievement and funding level is common in many countries and consequently poses a powerful dilemma for coaches and officials when choosing between an Olympic medal and continued or enhanced public funding on the one hand, and challenging a successful elite athlete suspected of using drugs on the other. The enthusiasm of the Australian Olympic Federation was, at that time, no greater than that of the AIS. The federation was deliberately slow in introducing random out-of-competition testing so as not to compromise athletes before the Olympic trials and also to enable them to ensure they were "clean" before testing commenced. Governing body and government determination to eradicate doping was further undermined by an acknowledgement that many other countries and, until recently, especially those in the communist bloc, had little commitment to drug-free sport. As was made clear in Chapter 2, there are currently similar concerns about the commitment of the Chinese sports authorities to anti-doping objectives.

The report of the senate inquiry was an indictment of the approach of Australian sports organisations towards anti-doping. The report criticised the testing regime because "there are major questions over the collection of urine samples, the selection of athletes for tests and the low frequency of testing".[1] Up to the time of the inquiry only 239 tests had been carried out and none had proved positive. The standard of administration of testing was also criticised on the grounds that athletes were able to provide a sample unchaperoned, and twenty athletes turned up to provide their sample up to thirty days after the forty-eight-hour deadline and incurred no penalty. The conclusions of the committee could hardly have been more damning. According to the committee, the institute's testing programme "was a response to outside pressures to be seen to be ' drug-free', rather than from any real concern for the need to strictly apply IOC guidelines to ensure the integrity of Australian sport and the health of its athletes. ... The committee believes that in many ways the AIS drug testing program was worse than having no drug testing program at all. It provided the protection of appearing to do something to prevent the use of drugs, but was conducted in such a manner that it may have been possible for athletes using drugs to claim that the program showed them to be drug free".[2]

The investigations of the Senate Committee marked a significant turning point in anti-doping policy in Australia. However, the reinvigoration of anti-doping policy was due to an intensification of government involvement and consequently at the cost of governing body autonomy. The main outcome of the inquiry was the establishment by law of the Australian Sports Drug

---

1. Ibid., p. 494.
2. Ibid., p. 495.

Agency (ASDA) in 1990 which was given the objective of reducing "the harm associated with the use of drugs in sport in order to promote the well-being of the individual and enhance the value of sport to society". ASDA's mission was supported by the role adopted by the Australian Sports Commission, a government agency, which required any governing body receiving public funds to comply with ASDA doping regulations. The impact of government intervention through ASDA has been dramatic, with the number of tests rising rapidly to over 2000 each year and covering almost fifty sports. Although tests are spread across a range of sports, those with a history of drug abuse are allocated a higher proportion of tests. Since the establishment of ASDA there has been a steady decline in the number of doping infractions and in the number of examples of "inadvertent use" of drugs by athletes. Part of the explanation for these trends probably lies in the success of the drug-testing programme, but there is also the concern that it may reflect the increasing sophistication of drug users who have moved on to some of the newer and less easily detected drugs. In general, the senate inquiry resulted in a considerable improvement in the effectiveness of anti-doping policy implementation and places Australia among the group of countries with the more reputable records on combating drug abuse. However, the cost of the improvement in compliance by athletes and their governing bodies has been a substantial increase in the involvement of government in the activities of voluntary bodies.

A similar pattern can be found in the United Kingdom except that the involvement of government dates from a much earlier phase of policy development. As early as the mid 1960s, the newly established Advisory Sports Council took an interest in the emerging issue of drug abuse by athletes. However, it was from the late 1980s that government intervention became more evident. In part the increase in government involvement was the result of frustration at the recalcitrance of a small number of governing bodies and the general lack of urgency of the sector to introduce more rigour and commitment to policy implementation and refinement. Government intervention was also stimulated by the increasing rumours of collusion in the undermining of drug testing by sports authorities. In general, the strategy of the government was to rely on exhortation and inducements to encourage governing bodies to take a more determined lead in the development and implementation of anti-doping measures. However, by the mid 1980s it was apparent that the pace of change was too slow for the government's liking. In 1985, the chair of the British Sports Council criticised governing bodies for dragging their feet on drug testing despite the fact that the cost of testing was underwritten completely by the Council. At about the same time that the disquiet within government was growing, a series of allegations was published in *The Times*, in December 1987, which claimed that coaches and officials were colluding in aiding athletes to avoid both testing and the publication of positive results. The allegations were subsequently investigated by a committee of inquiry instigated by the Amateur Athletic Association and chaired by the lawyer Peter Coni.[1] Although many of the more damaging allegations were rejected, the report created a strong impression that domestic governing bodies of sport were unprepared, if not simply unable, to respond effectively to the challenge of doping.

While the Coni report was published too late to have been a direct influence on government thinking, it certainly reinforced the conclusions that had already been drawn regarding the need to strengthen the anti-doping campaign through the adoption by the government of a more prominent role in policy implementation. A report co-authored by the sports minister, Colin Moynihan and the athlete, Sebastian Coe, in 1987, led, in 1988, to the establishment of the Doping Control Unit as an agency within the British Sports Council. The role of the unit was to provide information and develop educational material, but also to co-ordinate and conduct testing. The unit in effect took control of the technical aspects of testing and left the governing bodies with the responsibility for identifying those to be tested and dealing with positive results. The establishment of the unit came at the same time as the introduction of out-of-competition testing. As was the case in Australia, the pattern of policy development in the United Kingdom has resulted in a very similar testing regime and a greatly enhanced role for government and its agencies.

The pattern is little different in Canada where anti-doping policy in the 1970s and early 1980s was characterised by governing body inertia combined with governmental indifference until the dramatic positive drug test by Ben Johnson at the 1988 Olympics. The Dubin Inquiry that investigated the Johnson affair and the existing anti-doping policy was scathing in its description of a sports community at best unwilling to investigate the claims of widespread drug abuse voiced by a minority of coaches and officials, and at worst a community that actively colluded in the development of a drug-based elite sports culture. As in Australia and the United Kingdom, the outcome of the upsurge of government interest in the policy issue was the establishment of an anti-doping agency, the Canadian Centre for Drug-free Sport, which co-ordinated the testing programme and technical analysis, and also gave a clear lead to sports governing bodies on other aspects of policy implementation, including athlete selection and penalties to be applied to sportsmen and women guilty of doping infractions.

If the late 1980s can be characterised as a watershed in policy development which marked, in many countries, a substantial increase in government involvement in policy development and implementation, it is ironic that this was occurring at the same time that the elaborate state sports structures of the communist bloc in central and eastern Europe were disintegrating. In Europe, the collapse of communism ended a prolonged period of state

---

1. Amateur Athletics Association, "AAA Drug Abuse Report", (chair Peter Coni), London, AAA (1988).

dominated and manipulated sport best characterised by the maintenance of sham amateurism, but which touched all aspects of sport from the distortion of sporting opportunities in favour of the elite to the disadvantage of the mass of the population, on the one hand, "to the long term state production, testing, monitoring, and administering of performance-enhancing drugs in regard to athletes as young as seven and eight", on the other.[1] The year 1989 brought a rapid collapse of the communist state sports infrastructure and confronted governments and sports authorities with immense problems in refashioning a sports system that benefited the mass of the population and also attempted to retain some level of elite success. In many respects," ex-communist sport" faces an acute dilemma. The scaling down of the intensity of state control over sport provides an opportunity to rebuild a drug-free sports system, but the poverty of most of the former communist countries and the current priority among some to define rapidly a refashioned national identity makes the establishment of drug-free sport more difficult.

The pressures on sports administrators and athletes to acknowledge the legacy of the sports system of former communist countries is amply illustrated in the reunified Germany. Despite initial declarations that the East German sports system would be totally dismantled after reunification, the German Government has become increasingly ambivalent about some aspects of the East German system. At worst, condemnation of state-sponsored doping in the East was tempered by a deeply ambiguous attitude to doping among some athletes and coaches in the Federal Republic. According to Hoberman, "The enormous success of East German athletes at the 1976 Montreal Olympic Games produced a traumatic effect on the West German sports establishment that ended only with the collapse of the Communist state".[2] In late 1990, following a series of highly publicised and damaging revelations of doping in the former East Germany, but also in West Germany, an Independent Doping Commission was established supported by the government, the National Olympic Committee and the DSB (the German Sports Federation). While the commission found evidence of extensive doping in the former German Democratic Republic and evidence of less extensive but nonetheless significant doping in the Federal Republic of Germany, its conclusions were muted. In contrast to Australia and Canada, for example, the commission recommended leaving the resolution of the problem in the hands of sports authorities rather than advocating greater government involvement. More ambivalently, it recommended a doping amnesty thus legitimising the ratification of East German records as German national records. Finally, the commission's emphasis on the significance of elite sporting success for

---

1. Riordan, J., "Communist Sports Policy, The End of an Era", in *Chalip*, L., Johnson, A. & Stachura, L. *National Sports Policies, An International Handbook*, Westport, Conn., Greenwood Press (1996), p. 111.
2. Hoberman, J., *Mortal Engines, The Science of Performance and the Dehumanisation of Sport*, New York, The Free Press, p. 242.

nation-building in the new Germany provides the most likely reason for the commission's reluctance to challenge doping more forcefully. Germany's results at the Atlanta Olympic Games demonstrated the extent to which unified Germany relied on the children of the communist sports system. Of the total of 104 medals won, forty-eight were won by former East Germans: twelve of the twenty-two gold medals were also won by former East Germans. The significance of the contribution by East Germans to national success is illustrated by the fact that they account for only 21% of the total German population. However, as the evidence of systematic doping within the GDR has accumulated, the attitude of the German Government has hardened considerably with a series of prosecutions of coaches alleged to have caused "bodily harm to minors" through the administration of drugs. The government has also amended the statute of limitations to allow investigation of doping to continue until October 2000.

Maintaining the momentum

A central role in the development of sport in post-communist Europe has been played by the Council of Europe. Much of the responsibility for maintaining the momentum on anti-doping policy following the preparation of the convention lay with the monitoring group which has met annually since 1989. A significant amount of the work of the group has focused on a series of technical and legal aspects of policy development and implementation, but the work of the group also reflected the shift of emphasis away from treating doping as a discrete aspect of sports policy and towards seeing anti-doping policy as an integral element in a broader set of sports ethics. The work of the group complemented the increasing concern of the Council to identify and reinforce the ethical basis of sport and the positive contribution of sport to society in general and to the young in particular. In 1990 the Council, through the Comité Directeur pour le Développment du Sport (CDDS), published the conclusions of its debates on the responsibilities of parents and teachers in inculcating positive values towards drug-free competition. A year later a seminar was organised that focused on sports ethics and young people, and although concerned primarily with issues of fair play more generally, the debate had a deep resonance for those developing and promoting the anti-doping policy. The emphasis on ethical issues was reflected most strongly in the publication of the European Sports Charter in 1992 which took, as one of its aims, the commitment to "protect and develop the moral and ethical bases of sport (...) by safeguarding sport, sportsmen and women from (...) practices that are abusive or debasing, including the abuse of drugs". The Council adopted a Code of Sports Ethics in the same year which also emphasised the centrality of drug-free sport to the broader notion of fair play.

The elaboration of the political and ethical context for sport over the last ten years has been matched by a continuing refinement of testing procedures and technologies. The introduction of in-competition testing in the late 1960s, the development of GC/MS analytical techniques in the 1980s, and the introduction of out-of-competition testing in the late 1980s all represent quantum steps in testing procedures. However, it is also important to note the rapidity with which these developments have been matched by the drug abuser. As Voy notes, "The science of avoiding drug detection is probably as sophisticated today as the science of drug testing itself".[1] Voy cites two examples from 1988 when athletes, especially in field events, withdrew from competition because of the nature and timing of the testing procedures to be adopted. Competitions scheduled close to the date of the Olympic trials in the United States were especially vulnerable as drug-using athletes would still have been taking steroids. At the 1988 Pepsi Classic, scheduled a few weeks before the Olympic trials, the shot put and discus events had to be cancelled because so few athletes accepted the invitation to participate.[2] By the late 1980s, it was apparent that the effectiveness of out-of-competition testing was under threat because of the improved knowledge among drug abusers of the clearance time for drugs, combined with the practice of giving advance warning of an out-of-competition test. Advance notice testing which was common in many countries made a mockery of claims of rigour made by the advocates of out-of-competition testing. In some countries advance warning of up to a month might be given and, even where the period of notice was much shorter, the fact that the more sophisticated steroids could be flushed out of the system in under forty-eight hours meant that the drug abuser was under little real threat of identification. In the early 1990s a number of countries introduced no-notice testing, but the practice is far from the norm across all sports and countries. However, by the mid 1990s, of those countries that had introduced out-of-competition testing, 64% of tests were conducted with no notice and no country had an advance notice period of greater than forty-eight hours.

Conclusion

The relative novelty of the policy issue is compounded by two major factors, first the complexity of the issue and second its dynamic nature. The complexity can be illustrated in many ways, but one could simply point to the necessity to develop a policy which is effective at both domestic and international levels, which involves approximately thirty Olympic federations and a similar number of non-Olympic federations and which requires the co-operation of over one hundred or so governments which have a significant number of athletes participating in international competition. The dynamism of the policy area is best reflected in the constant, and largely successful, search on the part of drug-abusing athletes for new substances and practices which are more difficult to detect. One might also point to the global mobility of

1. Voy, R., op. cit., p. 93.
2. Ibid., p. 94.

athletes, to the ambivalence of many doctors and other professionals towards doping, and to the willingness of some governments to view international sporting success as a convenient resource in international relations.

An acknowledgement of the novelty, complexity and dynamism of the policy issue is important in any assessment of progress in developing a response to the problem of doping in sport. With this caveat in mind it would be fair to claim that much has been achieved if measured in terms of agreement on what to test for, what procedures to adopt in the administration of anti-doping policies, and how to deal with doping infractions. From a position in the early 1960s where those, admittedly few, federations concerned with drug abuse were developing separate lists of proscribed substances, there is now a strong consensus constructed around the IOC list which rapidly established itself as the benchmark. Indeed, one sign of the growing maturity of the policy discussions is that sports federations are beginning to refine the IOC list to meet the specific character and problems of their own sport. However, the content of the list is only significant if federations and countries intend to develop a programme of testing of which it is a part. Adopting the IOC or similar list does not in itself constitute an anti-doping policy. A much more tortuous process has been that of establishing a broad agreement on the process of anti-doping policy implementation. Progress has been painfully slow in reaching agreement on a large number of procedural questions including who to test, how many tests to conduct, the balance between in-competition and out-of-competition testing, the appropriate distribution of tests between sports, whether and how sampling officers should be trained and who should pay them and for their training, under what conditions should urine samples be collected, what constitutes the maintenance of an effective "chain of custody", which laboratories are suitable to undertake sample analysis, when should positive results be announced, when and under what circumstances is a positive result declared to be a doping infraction, and what appeals procedures are appropriate.

The difficulty of achieving agreement on procedural questions is amply illustrated by the history of penalties for doping infractions. The emerging consensus regarding penalties for the use of steroids appears to be for a two year ban for a first offence followed by a life ban for a subsequent offence. However, the fragility of this consensus is illustrated by the continuing debate among international federations and the periodic attempts by athletes to challenge the decisions of federations in the courts. On the positive side, there is a growing concern within federations to tailor the range of penalties to suit the characteristics of particular sports. For some sports, such as some disciplines in gymnastics, a two year ban for steroid use would represent exclusion from a substantial part of an athlete's career: for other sports, such as middle distance running, a two year ban would be far less damaging as the career tends to be longer. The concern to achieve a degree of equity between sports is hampered by a number of factors, not least of which is the periodic challenge to federation decisions in domestic courts. The increasing adoption of a two year ban for a first offence involving a major drug such as steroids is a retreat from an earlier preference for a four year ban and is due to the mounting of a successful legal challenge in the German courts and the threat of litigation elsewhere.

In addition to tracing the level of agreement on particular aspects of policy, the development of anti-doping policy could also be traced along four main dimensions, namely, clarification of policy focus, generation and maintenance of political commitment, technology development, and establishment of the necessary resource infrastructure. Table 6.3 (p. 150) provides a summary of change and indicates both the areas of progress, but also the areas where substantial difficulties remain.

As regards the clarity of policy focus, it is possible to trace the interweaving of a series of policy strands over the last forty years. One strand relates to the particular sports seen as most "at risk" and consequently acting as a focus for policy debates. In the 1950s and 1960s, cycling was the main source of concerns, followed in the 1970s by the throwing events and weightlifting: more recently, swimming and track events have been seen as the sports most vulnerable to drug users. The significance for policy makers of the association of the problem with particular sports is that each sport or cluster of sports generates distinct public perceptions. Doping infractions in cycling, as a largely professional sport, rarely generated the intensity of public condemnation as doping cases in the "amateur" sports of track and field. Similarly, doping in swimming and track events have generated a greater intensity of condemnation than doping in weightlifting and field events, possibly because the former sports are perceived as more truly symbolic of the Olympic virtues. A second strand in defining the current focus of policy is the steady shift from the athlete to the athlete's entourage and an increasingly common debate as to whether the athlete was best seen as the villain, victim or co-conspirator. The third policy strand is closely related to the previous theme and concerns the debate about the degree to which the domestic governing body should be held responsible for the drug abuse of its members. The international federations responsible for weightlifting and swimming have both considered suspending domestic governing bodies when breaches of doping regulations by their athletes are considered unacceptably high.

The second dimension to doping policy is the generation and maintenance of political commitment. In many respects the emergence of the issue of doping in sport and its transformation from a private issue to a public problem is a classic example of agenda-setting through crisis. Although there was an awareness of drug abuse in sport as a fringe aspect of the broader problem of social drug abuse, it was marginal to the concerns of anti-drug strategists largely because drug abuse in sport was seen as minor in extent, generally involving non-addictive drugs and substances that were legally available. In addition, there was, and remains, an understandable reluctance to add to the

149

Table 6.3 : The evolution of anti-doping policy

	Policy focus	Level and scope of support for anti-doping policy	Technological development	Development of implementation infrastructure
1950s	Highly generalised, but concern is focused on one or two sports such as cycling.	Debate largely confined to specialists within specific sports and a small number of sports	Little specifically directed at drug testing in sport.	Almost none.
1960s	Early definitions of the problem are produced but are confused.	Widespread collusion among governments in doping, for example in the former GDR and Soviet Union. Still only a minority of major federations involved in anti-doping activity.	Testing refined for amphetamines.	Limited in-competition testing, but few international federations had anti-doping regulations. Few countries had laws relating to the misuse of drugs in sport. IOC Medical Commission (re)-established in 1967.
1970s	Focus on amateur rather than professional sport; some concern with addictive drugs in professional sport; start of a process of locating doping within the broader values of sport, e.g. "Sport for All".	Most governments at best lukewarm in their support for anti-doping; others ambivalent towards emerging anti-doping policy. Wide variation in the level of commitment to anti-doping among federations.	Testing developed for narcotic analgesics and stimulants. Later, in 1976, testing developed for steroids by radioimmunoassay.	Increase in testing, but still unreliable consequently few positives declared. IAAF Medical Committee established in 1972. IAAF & IOC accreditation of laboratories in mid 1970s. Still many weaknesses in procedure e.g. regarding the "chain of custody".
1980s	Shift of emphasis from deterrence alone to deterrence plus education.	Series of major scandals prompting sharp increase in government and federation interest.	Testing available for caffeine. Testing also available for beta-blockers and blood-doping in 1985 and for diuretics in 1987. GC/MS testing for steroids in late 1980s.	Mid to late 1980s increase in government legislation against steroid trafficking; 1985 laboratory re-accreditation by the IOC introduced. Out-of-competition testing introduced in late 1980s.
1990s	Increasing concern to locate doping within an articulation of the ethics of sport; shift (or broadening) of focus from the athlete alone to the athlete and entourage (i.e. penalties for coaches, doctors and even for domestic governing bodies); debate about athletes as victims or villains. Increasing concern with broad policy harmonisation.	Increasing sophistication of debates within the federations and the IOC, and also within governmental organisations such as the Council of Europe. Increasing awareness of the complexity of the issue leading both to greater commitment by some policy actors and to greater uncertainty and weakening of resolve among others.	Testing for growth hormone by 2000	IOC established Court of Arbitration. Increase in the number of international forums in which to discuss doping policy (e.g. Permanent World Conference on Doping, Nordic Group, CE and EU). Increase in government-funded research into drug testing.

burden of anti-drug policing by criminalising a new set of drugs and users especially when there was not the extensive association between sports-drug use and crimes such as smuggling, street crime and violence. For most international federations and domestic governing bodies, commitment to anti-doping has been slow to develop partly because of a reluctance to acknowledge the problem as specific to sport, partly due to an awareness of the resource implications of developing and implementing an anti-doping strategy, and partly, for some federations at least, the result of an unwillingness to recognise doping as a challenge to sports ethics. For some domestic governing bodies there is an additional motive for remaining unenthusiastic about anti-doping, namely a fear of alienating star athletes on whom they depend for the success of sports competitions. However, it is not just governing bodies that are reluctant to name those who produce positive test results. In late 1996 it was alleged that the IOC had failed to announce four positive test results, in addition to the two that were reported at the time of the Atlanta games.

With some notable exceptions the ambivalence of many federations towards doping was a reflection of the often highly ambiguous attitude of governments to the issue. The blatant hypocrisy, for much of the post-war period, of the governments in the communist countries of eastern and central Europe was matched by the casual indifference of many, if not most, governments in non-communist industrialised countries. The level of state-supported doping has declined but there have been accusations of state complicity in doping directed towards the People's Republic of China. Until the series of positives at the Perth World Swimming Championships in January 1998, it had been thought that the Chinese Government had become aware of the damage to the PRC's reputation and to the poor prospects of hosting future major track and field events that resulted from its weak stand on anti-doping. That three Chinese athletes tested positive in early 1997 for steroids might have suggested that nothing much had changed, but the fact that they were identified by the domestic governing body rather than by international federation testing officers indicated a possible change of attitude. However, the Perth episodes have once again raised serious doubts about the sincerity of the Chinese authorities' protestations of commitment to drug-free sport. For most countries, policy making was scandal driven, with the stimulus for many governments being the desire to maintain the utility of international sport as a tool of foreign policy and general positive public relations. It remains to be seen whether the recent scandals will prompt the Chinese authorities to demonstrate a stronger commitment to anti-doping, if for no other reason than to retain the diplomatic utility of international sport.

The third dimension of policy relates to the pace of technology development. The IOC has generally been reluctant to place a substance on its list of banned drugs until a reliable testing method had been identified. The development of radioimmunoassay analysis in the mid 1970s enabled steroids to be added to the IOC list and the more recent refinement of gas chromatography/mass spectrometry analysis proved to be a major development in the detection of traces of steroids, forcing drug users to allow a much longer clearance period. Although technological and analytical developments have been significant, there is a major concern that the techniques of drug detection will be unable to keep pace with the increasing sophistication of newer drugs and especially those that enhance or replicate the normal chemistry of the body. A major issue for the success of current anti-doping policy and also for the credibility of future policy is the ability of federations and governments to fund research into detection techniques. Finally, there has been considerable progress in the development of an infrastructure to support policy implementation. On the one hand, the establishment and maintenance of a network of accredited laboratories is of major importance in reducing the likelihood of legal challenge to the laboratory analysis. However, the cost of maintaining an IOC-accredited laboratory continues to escalate as the analytic techniques increase in sophistication and greater sensitivity of measurement is needed. The distribution of laboratories is uneven, with most being located in Europe and North America, and with there being little likelihood of poorer countries ever having an accredited laboratory. The uneven distribution of laboratories also means that research into testing techniques is also confined to a small group of countries. A further element of the policy infrastructure is the regulatory framework operated by federations and governments. Although there is less diversity of regulatory practice than ten or twenty years ago, there is still substantial variation between federations on many aspects of sampling procedure and also variations between governments on matters such as the importation, sale and possession of steroids and the willingness of domestic courts to support bans for drug use.

In highlighting the weaknesses in current anti-doping policy implementation, one should not lose sight of the achievements. In a relatively short period of time a basic policy infrastructure has been put in place and the issue of doping in sport is prominent on the agendas of federations and an increasing number of governments, many of whom have allocated considerable sums of public money to support anti-doping policy. It is probably fair to conclude that the initial stage of policy development is coming to an end and a new agenda of issues is emerging which will test the capacity of the international sporting community to maintain the policy commitment and momentum. At the forefront of the new agenda of issues is the question of policy harmonisation both across federations and sports and also across countries.

Chapter 7

Policy harmonisation: problems and prospects

Given the major differences between individual sports and between the importance given to sport in different countries, it might be considered surprising that more sports bodies do not challenge the current priority being given to the objective of harmonisation. Yet the questioning of the objective is relatively slight. Some established professional sports have argued that they should not be expected to adhere to the same doping rules as "amateur" sports. Similarly, some professional sportsmen and women have argued that sport is their living and that they should be allowed more leeway in the range of permissible drugs, particularly those used to control pain. Occasional challenges to harmonisation are also heard from the non-Olympic sports which argue that it is both unnecessary and unfair to impose IOC standards on non-Olympic sports. Despite sporadic questioning of moves towards harmonisation, the issue has generally prompted few debates and even fewer objections. Yet far from the absence of debate being a sign that harmonisation is uncontentious, it is more a sign that harmonisation is still at its very earliest stages of development and is, as yet, not perceived as a threat to organisational autonomy. More seriously, it is likely that there are a number of key organisations that have, at best, a lukewarm commitment to harmonisation and believe that it will remain an aspiration rather than a reality for a long time to come.

Part of the basis for the belief that extensive harmonisation is remote is a continuing ambiguity concerning what is understood by the objective of harmonisation. It is possible to argue that over the last thirty years there has been significant movement towards harmonisation especially when compared to many other attempts at obtaining international policy uniformity, such as those in the areas of environmental protection and free trade. In major aspects of policy such as definitions of doping, the list of banned substances and practices, and penalties, there is considerable agreement. If one considers the question of harmonisation as a spectrum with agreement on broad principles at one end and uniformity of detail at the other, it is appropriate to ask how far along the spectrum towards detailed uniformity the sought-for harmonisation lies. Underlying this question are others, such as which aspects of doping policy it is more important to harmonise than others. There is also the interesting question of where the source of the demand for greater harmonisation lies. It is possible to identify two major sources, one with government and the other with sports organisations. Whether the two sets of organisations share a common perception of harmonisation is part of the subject of this chapter.

The primary stimulus for the current emphasis on harmonisation is the recognition of the global character of elite sports circuits and the high level of international mobility of elite athletes. There is little point in the government and domestic governing bodies of sport in one particular country having a clear set of regulations regarding doping if their elite athletes do not train in their home country nor participate in competition in that country. There are plenty of examples of world class athletes, particularly from outside Europe, that have little or no contact with the anti-doping regime of their home country. Because the major cycling competitions are in Europe there are, for example, few world class Australian cyclists who compete or train extensively in Australia. Much the same can be said regarding the top class soccer players from South America, and increasingly Africa, who spend most of their careers in Europe. Given the multiplicity of sources of legitimate anti-doping regulation and the global nature of modern elite sport, it is important that there is maximum uniformity of regulations so that drug abusers are not able to exploit differences and inconsistencies between countries, domestic governing bodies and international federations. The clearest motives for harmonisation are first, equity of treatment of elite athletes and second, the increasing concern to prevent a successful legal challenge to the decisions of international federations.

The problems of inconsistency

The case involving Katrin Krabbe is a valuable illustration of the problems that can arise from inconsistency between rule-making authorities. In January 1992, three German athletes, Katrin Krabbe, Silke Möller and Grit Breur, were tested at their winter training camp in South Africa. The out-of-competition tests were requested by the German athletic federation, Deutscher Leichtathletik Verband (DLV), and were carried out by the South African Amateur Athletic Federation. The analysis, at the IOC-accredited laboratory in Cologne, revealed that the urine samples were identical. The athletes were suspected of breaching regulations concerning the manipulation of samples. The decision of the DLV presidium was to suspend the athletes for a breach of regulations. However, the athletes appealed on a number of grounds including that the DLV lacked the authority to conduct out-of-competition tests and that the sanctions imposed were not allowable under the terms of the DLV constitution. The subsequent review of the decision by the DLV Legal Committee found in favour of the athletes and the suspension was lifted. The investigation of the two decisions of the DLV by the IAAF concluded that the Legal Committee had been correct. The key weakness in the DLV presidium decision was the fact that the doping rules of the association had not been incorporated into the constitution of the federation but were contained in a separate document. This being the case, it was accepted that under German law the testing lacked constitutional validity and no legitimate penalty could be imposed. The lesson to be learned from the episode was that "In order for each (inter)national federation to be able to conduct effective anti-doping controls, the authority of the (inter)national federation to conduct such testing should be firmly supported by a provision to this effect in the constitution of the (inter)national federation in question".[1] In other words, the domestic governing body to which the athlete belongs must explicitly recognise the authority of the domestic federations of other countries and that of the international federation to conduct tests on its members.

Krabbe's renewed eligibility to compete was short-lived as she tested positive for steroids in July the same year. The IAAF announced the doping infraction in August and the DLV imposed a four year suspension on the athlete. However, Krabbe successfully undermined the DLV decision by threatening to challenge the decision in the German courts on the grounds that the scale of the penalty was too severe. Facing the prospect of a potentially costly legal battle, the DLV reduced the penalty to one year's suspension. If the lesson of the previous episode was to ensure consistency between federations, the lesson of this case was to attempt to achieve greater consistency between the scale of penalties deemed appropriate by the international federation and those accepted as fair by domestic legal systems.

Further demonstration of the need for greater harmonisation came from a case concerning the Australian athlete Martin Vinnicombe. Vinnicombe, a cyclist, was tested in Canada at the request of the Australian Sports Drug Agency (ASDA) in May 1991. At first glance the procedures were followed meticulously: ASDA had sent a letter of authorisation to the Canadian authorities and when the sample was taken Vinnicombe signed a declaration of satisfaction with the procedures. The samples were analysed at an IOC-accredited laboratory in Montreal where traces of the steroid stanozolol were found, whereupon Vinnicombe was suspended from competition for two years, a period consistent with the rules of both the domestic governing body and the international federation. As de Pencier noted, "Vinnicombe never denied that he had in fact used stanozolol".[2] However, this did not prevent him challenging the suspension in the Australian courts on the grounds that "the test results ought to be invalidated because of the variations between doping control set out in the ASDA Act and ASDA Regulations and as set out in the Canadian Doping Control Standard Operating Procedures".[3] The judge in the federal court suggested mediation with Bob Ellicott, a former minister responsible for sport, acting as mediator. Ellicott ultimately found that, although it was clear that Vinnicombe had taken steroids, the sanctions

---

1. Council of Europe and European Union "Clean Sport Guide", (1995), Section B, module 8, p. 3.
2. de Pencier, J., "Law and Athlete Drug Testing in Canada", *Marquette Sports Law Journal*, Vol. 4.2, (1994), p. 295.
3. Ibid., p. 296.

imposed on him were invalid because the strict ASDA procedures for doping control had not been followed.[1] Bearing in mind that this incident took place only three years after a major overhaul of the doping control procedures in the wake of the AIS scandal, it demonstrates the difficulty of ensuring that the regulations governing drug testing are watertight and fulfil the purpose for which they were drafted.

The globalisation of sports competition circuits and the increasing geographical mobility of elite sportsmen and women has been matched and stimulated by a rapid commercialisation of sport and the growing wealth of elite athletes. These developments have been paralleled by a greater willingness among athletes to initiate legal proceedings to defend their income if not their innocence! The increased litigiousness of athletes has prompted a high level of nervousness among governing bodies, resulting in a welcome enhancement in attention to the detail of the testing procedures but also a reluctance to take action against athletes suspected of a doping infraction. The readiness of athletes to seek damages against governing bodies and federations and the financial weakness of most sports organisations provides added urgency for the achievement of harmonisation. Without greater harmonisation, there is a risk that doping policy will atrophy as the evident tentativeness among sports authorities gives way to a paralysis based on fear of making decisions vulnerable to legal challenge.

Any progress towards closer harmonisation of policy involves close co-operation between governing bodies of sport and governments. The engagement of governments with the issue of doping is not just part of the general trend towards greater government intervention in sport in modern society, it is also a consequence of the particular character of the issue of doping involving, as it does, the use of many substances that are already illegal or else tightly regulated. It is, therefore, not surprising that the impetus for harmonisation should have two sources, one within governmental organisations and the other among sports organisations. Governmental efforts to improve harmonisation centre on the activity of the Council of Europe while the IOC is the focus for discussions among the international federations.

The international response to doping and the role of the Council of Europe

In general, the division of function between federations and governments is that the former are responsible for determining, *inter alia*, the list of banned substances and practices, selecting athletes for testing, the penalties for doping infractions and the management of any appeals system. In some countries, federations also have responsibility for determining the number of tests and the balance between in-competition and out-of-competition testing, but in others these responsibilities rest with government. Governments tend to

---

1. Ibid., p. 296.

take responsibility for funding the testing regime and providing a legal context for the prohibition of certain drugs. In addition, governments are often heavily involved in underwriting the cost of research into anti-doping methods, providing training for sampling officers, and providing elements of the administrative infrastructure for doping control. Broadly speaking, governments provide important elements of the administrative, financial and legal framework within which the anti-doping policies of the federations and domestic governing bodies function.

The growth in concern with policy harmonisation is best indicated by the steady involvement of governments in international discussions regarding doping. Governments have played a significant role as initiators of international forums and multilateral and bilateral links which provide opportunities for the discussion and monitoring of anti-doping policy. The Council of Europe is the primary example, but both the European Union and Unesco have provided occasional arenas for discussions about drug abuse by athletes. In addition to these permanent forums a number of governments, usually through their anti-doping agency, have entered into bilateral agreements, often involving the sharing of expertise, research, training of personnel, and testing of partner countries' athletes. The bilateral agreement between Australia and China is a good example of an agreement designed to pool expertise and research, and to develop training programmes in doping control. Similar bilateral agreements exist between Norway and China, France and Germany, Canada and Cuba and also between Canada and France. The Nordic Anti-doping Agreement links a range of northern European countries including Denmark, Iceland, Finland, Sweden and Norway and provides not only for the testing of signatories' athletes, but also the sharing of expertise and research. In addition, the Nordic group of countries are committed to harmonisation of rules and penalties as well as to common action to limit the availability of drugs. The Nordic Agreement was opened for signature in 1996 with Germany being one of the first countries to be invited to sign. The more recent Baltic Anti-doping Agreement is intended to fulfil a broadly similar function within its region. Since 1989 there has been a series of permanent world conferences on doping, providing an opportunity largely for government anti-doping agencies and specialist groups such as scientists and doctors to exchange information, but also involving representatives from sports organisations.

Finally, there is a group of countries that subscribe to the International Anti-Doping Agreement (formerly the Memorandum of Understanding Group) which shares similar objectives to the Nordic group, namely the mutual testing of member's athletes, shared research and progress on harmonisation. The membership of the group currently includes Australia, Canada, New Zealand, Norway, Sweden and the United Kingdom. France was a member until recently. The primary focus of the efforts of the group is on harmonisation and specifically the need to agree objective quality standards as a secure basis for mutual trust and confidence building. To this end, a four year plan (adopted in 1995) is in place which aims to "ensure the development and harmonisation of the domestic programmes of the signatories and thus by example of good practice, positively influence the international sporting community". The main vehicle for achieving this aim is through the development of a set of protocols for the doping control process which meet the thresholds for such standards set by the International Standards Organisation (ISO). The intention of the group is to produce a quality manual that covers all the major stages of the doping control process, from the selection and notification of athletes for doping control through sample analysis to hearings, sanctions and appeals. The draft standard is intended to be available for adoption towards the year 2000.

While it is true that many intergovernmental agreements can be a substitute for action or are initiated because of broader diplomatic imperatives, the pattern of agreements that now exist, with the Council of Europe's Anti-doping Convention at its heart, provides an important element of the infrastructure for policy development and implementation. Forty-one states have signed the Council of Europe convention, of which all but seven have ratified the convention and brought it into force (see Appendix C).[1] Interestingly the Council deliberately and unusually left the word "European" out of the title of the convention in order to make it clear that there was no geographical restriction and in the hope that the convention would become a global standard.

The driving force behind the implementation of the convention has been the Anti-doping Convention Monitoring Group which meets annually and operates through a series of working parties responsible for research, education and information, legislative measures and finally, technical co-operation. Some of the recent topics and projects undertaken by the working groups are tightly focused on current problems such as the development of standard procedures for blood sampling, the interpretation of testosterone/epitestosterone ratios, and the applicability of the convention to the non-sports use of prohibited substances. Other topics are much more broadly focused on issues associated with harmonisation and include the development of an education and information folder, *The Clean Sports Guide*, which aims to provide guidance on best practices in doping control, and the sanctions that should be taken with regard to an athlete's entourage following a doping infraction. However, even where the working parties are dealing with tightly focused issues, they function within the context of three overlapping and dominant concerns of the monitoring group, namely harmonisation, information dissemination and organisational networking.

At the first meeting of the monitoring group, it was agreed that a report from each contracting partner and observer would provide an annual report on domestic developments in anti-doping policy. The exchange of information

---

1. As of 28 October 1998.

through the system of annual reports has identified many of the issues that have become subjects for working group discussion. If the exchange of information is one obvious prerequisite for harmonisation then another is the construction of an effective interorganisational network for the dissemination of information and the discussion of policy. The greatest success of the monitoring group has been in consolidating membership within the new post-communist Europe and in extending contacts beyond the regional catchment area of the Council of Europe. Among the most recent signatories to the Anti-doping Convention are a number of countries of central and eastern Europe including Croatia, the Czech Republic, Estonia, Latvia, and the Russian Federation. Outside Europe, both Australia and Canada have ratified the convention and a range of other countries including the United States, Peru and Brazil, and most recently China and South Africa, have participated in the discussions of the monitoring group.

The monitoring group has also been relatively successful in building links with other governmental bodies such as Unesco, the World Health Organisation and the European Union. Although the leading role of the Council of Europe is now fairly secure among governmental bodies this has not always been the case. One of the early concerns of the monitoring group was the announcement by Unesco's Sports Committee that it intended to prepare an international instrument against doping in sport barely a year after the Council had agreed its own convention. However, Unesco was persuaded not to pursue its own convention and within a few years the Unesco committee was actively encouraging its members to sign the Council's convention, helped no doubt by the fact that the Council representative from Germany, Peter Glass, was also chair of the Unesco committee. A similarly broadly co-operative relationship has evolved between the Council and the European Union. In 1991, when the European Union meeting of health ministers proposed a code of conduct relating to doping, an invitation to participate in discussions was extended by the Union to the monitoring group. In general, the discussions of European Union Ministers for Sport are fairly closely informed by the work of the Council of Europe on sports matters. However, this does not prevent occasions when there has been the risk of duplication of work, as in 1994 when the European Parliament passed a resolution on doping and sport which, if implemented in full, would have overlapped substantially with the Council's convention. More recently, the Council and the European Union have co-operated closely on the production of the education and training pack, *The Clean Sports Guide*, for distribution among federations and domestic governing bodies. Finally, in recent years links have also been made between the Education Working Party of the Monitoring Group and the World Health Organisation which published in 1993 a major report on doping and sport.[1]

---

1. World Health Organisation, *Drug Use and Sport, Current Issues and Implications for Public Health*, Geneva, WHO, 1993.

Where the group has perhaps been less successful is in bringing sports organisations such as the IOC and the major federations into the network. The involvement of the IOC has been generally consistent and its representatives have on occasions made significant contributions to the work of the group. However, the committee seems to be content to provide encouragement for the work of the Council of Europe and to maintain a watching brief on the activities of the monitoring group rather than acknowledge the Council as the primary policy-making forum for public authorities and thereby sacrifice its own claims to policy leadership. A similar relationship exists between the international federations and the monitoring group. Although there is a clear awareness on the part of the governmental representatives and on the part of those from the federations that they share many fundamental concerns and objectives, there is also an acute wariness felt by the federations that control over their sports may be irretrievably undermined if policy leadership on anti-doping is ceded too readily to governments. For example, some federations are unhappy with national anti-doping authorities carrying out drug tests at federation competitions without consultation and argue that this was interference in their sphere of responsibility and that they would not consider themselves bound by the outcome of any result from a national anti-doping agency. One of the federations representing a major team sport has expressed a reluctance to take a greater responsibility for the conduct of out-of-competition testing, arguing that the workload would be too great. Given that the sport is one of the more affluent this is a surprising and worrying claim, but one that reflects the growing tensions within an increasingly commercialised sport where leagues, clubs, players and their domestic governing bodies are jockeying for control over the sport.

A different, but equally significant, objection to harmonisation was expressed by the representative of another major sport who, in response to a challenge that the federation had not yet subscribed to the 1994 Lausanne Agreement with the IOC concerning harmonisation, argued that it wished to retain its own schedule of sanctions which are generally lighter than those supported by the IOC, partly on the grounds that heavy sanctions breached the convicted athlete's "right to work". Although the record of this second federation in developing and implementing an anti-doping strategy is stronger than that of the federation referred to in the first example, both federations share a common concern to protect their autonomy, not just in relation to perceived encroachment by governments and government organisations such as the Council of Europe, but also in relation to other sports bodies such as the IOC.

The discussion of anti-doping policy in general and co-operation over harmonisation in particular is largely taking place in two arenas, one centred on governmental forums, especially the Council of Europe, and the other centred on sports organisations, particularly the IOC and the IAAF. Contact between the two clusters of interests is limited and characterised on the part of governments by a degree of scepticism about the level of commitment to anti-doping among federations, and a corresponding wariness on the part of sports federations that governments are seeking to undermine their control over their sports. The reluctance among key sports federations and organising bodies such as the IOC to become too closely integrated into the agenda of the Council of Europe and other governmental bodies is paralleled by a degree of mutual suspicion among federations which makes inter-federation co-operation, at times, difficult to achieve. If sports organisations are to prevent the anti-doping agenda being set by governments, then they need to be able to assert their control of the issue. Unfortunately, not only is there a significant degree of mutual suspicion between federations due to increasing competition for talented sportsmen and women, sponsorship, government support, and television revenue, but there is also a much more serious division between the federations on the one hand and the IOC on the other. Recently, the IAAF made it clear that it did not intend to recognise the Court of Arbitration for Sport in Lausanne as superior to its own arbitration panel. Furthermore, IAAF Secretary-General Istvan Gyulai expressed fundamental reservations about IOC claims to anti-doping policy leadership, arguing that "The IOC acts like a world government, but we do not want to be dominated in this way".[1] In addition, there is frequently tension within the Olympic movement over the division of sponsorship and television income arising from the Olympic Games.

Aware of the risk of losing the initiative in the formation of anti-doping policy, the IOC and the major federations have made a belated attempt to address the issue of harmonisation. However, progress so far has been limited. In 1995 the Council of Europe published an evaluation of the status of harmonisation among the federations[2] based on the collection of raw data by the British Sports Council's Doping Control Unit.[3] The conclusion of the report, prepared by Emile Vrijman, the Dutch representative on the Council's monitoring group, drew attention to a catalogue of weaknesses in the anti-doping rules of the major sports and highlighted the lack of harmonisation in a number of important areas of policy.

There have been a number of attempts, mainly in the mid to late 1980s, to achieve greater harmonisation of anti-doping rules among the federations and between the federations and the IOC. The most recent attempt was in January 1994 when a meeting, which included the IOC along with the organisations representing the summer and winter Olympic federations, decided to "unify their respective anti-doping rules and procedures".[4]

---

1. Quoted in *Sport Intern*, Vol. 29.ii, 1997, p. 6.
2. Vrijman, E.N., *Harmonisation, Can it Ever Really be Achieved?*, Strasbourg, Council of Europe, 1995.
3. Doping Control Unit, Sports Council, *Directory of Anti-doping Regulations of International Sports Federations*, 2nd edn., London, Sports Council, 1993.
4. Ibid., p. 5.

Vrijman's review was indeed timely as it was based on the anti-doping rules in force in 1993 and consequently provides a clear indication of the scale of challenge facing the IOC. Vrijman analysed the anti-doping rules of fifty-four international federations, paying special attention to their rules regarding the definition of doping; the list of banned drugs and methods of doping; forms of doping control; laboratory arrangements; penalties; recognition of sanctions imposed by other sports bodies; the right to a hearing; and the treatment of minor procedural mistakes. Apart from assessing the extent of harmonisation between the rules of the federations when compared to the anti-doping rules of the IOC, Vrijman's analysis was also concerned with assessing the extent to which federation rules were secure from legal challenge. In 1997 the United Kingdom's Sports Council's Ethics and Anti-doping Directorate published the third edition of its survey of current anti-doping regulations therefore providing useful data on the progress that has been made in the four years since the Lausanne Agreement.[1]

As should be evident from the discussion of definitions of doping in Chapter 5 and Chapter 6, there is no easy, let alone legally secure, answer to the question "What is doping in sport?". Charles Dubin argued that a definition was "impossible to achieve"[2] and quoted approvingly Sir Arthur Gold's comment that "to define doping is, if not impossible, at best extremely difficult, and yet everyone who takes part in competitive sport or who administers it knows exactly what it means. The definition lies not in words but in integrity of character".[3] While many would sympathise with the sentiments expressed by Dubin and Gold, a workable definition of doping is essential given the accelerating rate of legal challenge to the decisions of federations on doping infractions. "Integrity of character" provides the moral basis for the anti-doping policy but it is the words used to express that morality that will be scrutinised by lawyers. The importance of a clearly worded definition was reinforced by the judge who heard the case brought by Sandra Gasser against the IAAF in which she challenged their definition of doping as one of strict liability. The judge defended the IAAF definition and referred approvingly to the IAAF representative's concern that "if a defence of moral innocence were open, the floodgates would be opened and the IAAF's attempts to prevent drug taking by athletes would be rendered futile".[4] Mark Gay, in a presentation to the 4th Permanent World Conference on Anti-Doping in Sport, provided ample support for a definition based on strict liability by demonstrating the flaws in a wide range of definitions that were based on

---

1. Ethics and Anti-Doping Directorate, United Kingdom Sports Council, *Directory of Anti-doping Regulations of International Sports Federations*, 3rd. edn., London, UK Sports Council, 1997.
2. Dubin, C.L., "Commission of Inquiry into the use of drugs and banned practices intended to increase athletic performance", Ottawa, Canadian Government Publishing Centre, 1990.
3. Quoted in Dubin, op. cit., p. 78.
4. Gay, M., "Constitutional Aspects of Testing for Prohibited Substances", London, unpublished paper, no date.

criteria such as "intent" and "use in competition" rather than being based on the simple presence of banned substances in the urine or blood sample.[1] Vrijman reports Gay's advice that all federations should make doping an offence not dependent on proving an intention to cheat but rather based on strict liability. The IAAF is one of a small but growing number of federations that have adopted a "strict liability" definition. Writing in 1995 and using the IAAF definition as the benchmark, Vrijman reviewed the definitions of thirty-three other federations and found first, that all of them had definitions that were potentially vulnerable to legal challenge and second, that there was very little uniformity between sports. Many sports, such as squash and badminton, did not provide a definition of doping, while others included a sentence in their rules that associated them with the IOC rules on doping. Of those that did provide a definition, many were unclear and confused and, as mentioned earlier, vulnerable to legal challenge. In the four years since the collection of the data that Vrijman used, there has been some progress in amending anti-doping rules to make them less vulnerable to legal challenge. A small number of federations, including those for gymnastics and ice hockey, have adopted definitions similar to that used by the IAAF, but the vast majority have left their definitions unrevised. There is, despite the case quoted by Gay, growing doubt regarding the value of a "strict liability" definition, particularly in the United States. In 1995 the swimmer, Jessica Foschi, tested positive for the anabolic steroid mesterolone and was penalised under the rules of the international federation (FINA). She appealed against the penalty to the American Arbitration Association (AAA), the body prescribed under the terms of the United States Amateur Sports Act 1978. The AAA was emphatic in its rejection of the FINA decision and the application of the concept of "strict liability". The arbitrators argued that : "Having concluded that the claimant and all those connected with her are innocent and without fault, we unanimously conclude that the imposition of any sanction on the claimant so offends our deeply rooted and historical concepts of fundamental fairness so as to be arbitrary and capricious".[2] Similar rejections of the concept of strict liability have been provided by the Swiss courts and the legal committee of the German track and field federation with the latter arguing that "the maxim *nulla poena sine culpa* (no penalty without fault) has the

---

1. A definition based on "strict liability" would mean that a doping offence had been committed if a prohibited substance is present in an athlete's urine sample irrespective of whether the drug was taken knowingly or whether the drug was capable of enhancing performance. The IAAF definition of doping is as follows : "The offence of doping takes place when either (i) a prohibited substance is found to be present within an athlete's body tissue or fluids ; or (ii) an athlete uses or takes advantage of a prohibited technique ; or (iii) an athlete admits having used or taken advantage of a prohibited substance or prohibited technique" (IAAF Handbook 1992-93, Rule 55). According to Wise the "strict liability" definition means that an athlete can be found guilty of a doping infraction "without the sports governing body proving culpable intent, knowledge or fault ; or without the athlete being allowed to prove he or she was faultless" (Wise, A.N., "Strict liability" drug rules of sports governing bodies, in *New Law Journal*, 2 August, 1996, p. 1161).
2. Ibid., p. 1161.

status of a constitutional principle. Since the principle of the State Rechtsstaalichkeit is infringed, the corresponding provision in that case is grossly unfair and thus unenforceable".[1]

Vrijman found greater consistency regarding the adoption of a common list of banned substances and practices. Most federations have adopted the IOC list, although eight out of thirty-eight had adopted a specific, earlier list rather than the current list. Where there are variations they tend to be relatively minor modifications of the IOC list and often involve the specification of additional drugs that have a particular relevance to their sport. For example, the motor sport federation, Fédération Internationale du Sport Automobile (FISA), adds alcohol and marijuana to the IOC list of banned substances. In contrast the federation responsible for basketball, Fédération Internationale de Basketball Amateur (FIBA), varies the IOC list by allowing the use of beta-blockers. The results suggest that there is a minority of federations that are examining the IOC list and making minor modifications to ensure that it is appropriate to the specific requirements of their sport. However, there is also the strong suspicion that there is a number of federations that adopt the IOC list out of convenience rather than as a result of an analysis of the appropriateness of the IOC list to the particular characteristics of their sport. Adopting the IOC list of banned substances and practices is by far the easiest aspect of developing and implementing an anti-doping policy. Between 1993 and 1997 there had been some movement towards greater uniformity around the IOC list. Five sports, including bobsleigh, squash and shooting, had amended their rules by including a specific reference to the IOC list. In general the amendments made by the five federations involved the replacement of their own list of banned substances and practices with the current IOC list. As mentioned earlier, it is unclear whether the increasing standardisation of anti-doping regulations around the IOC list represents a recognition of the universal applicability of the list or a convenient response by federations seeking to shelter under the authority of the IOC, irrespective of the appropriateness of the list to their sport.

Much the same can be said for the relative uniformity among federations in their use of IOC-accredited laboratories for the analysis of samples. The fact that an increasing majority of federations use IOC-accredited laboratories provides little evidence of the extent of commitment to anti-doping policy. Agreeing to have samples analysed by IOC-accredited laboratories imposes few significant obligations. What matters more is the commitment to carry out a sufficient number of tests to make the analysis worthwhile.

One of the most pronounced trends in recent years has been the extension of testing into the out-of-competition period. Begun in the mid 1980s, and given a boost as a result of the Ben Johnson case, the extension of

---

1. Ibid., p1162.

out-of-competition testing is a priority of the signatories to the Lausanne Agreement. At the time of the second survey of anti-doping regulations in 1993, only sixteen out of fifty-four sports operated both in-competition and out-of-competition testing, indicating the scale of the problem that the supporters of the Lausanne Agreement faced. Moreover some thirty-eight federations would have needed to change their rules in order to introduce out-of-competition testing. By the time of the third survey in 1997 there had been a significant increase, from sixteen to twenty-five, in the number of federations undertaking in- and out-of-competition testing. Among the sports that had changed their rules were netball, squash, taekwondo, and cycling. However, it needs to be borne in mind that the balance between in- and out-of-competition testing will, of necessity, vary between sports with some sports with a very long season, such as soccer, understandably being less convinced of the value of out-of-competition tests. This still leaves a large number of sports, such as triathlon, wrestling, and bobsleigh, which have a closed season and which are comparable to those sports where steroid use is well known. In relation to the balance between in- and out-of-competition testing, one would need to apply a more subtle measure of harmonisation than mere uniformity. Unfortunately, the majority of federations are still some way from harmonisation on this aspect of policy whether one is expecting uniformity or a more sophisticated interpretation of the objective.

Many similar points may be made regarding the basis on which athletes are selected for testing and the number of athletes that are selected for testing. On the one hand, given the individual characteristics of each sport one should not expect uniformity : on the other hand, an analysis of the regulations of the federations suggests that while most sports have a selection process that is derived (albeit loosely in some cases) from the character of the sport, some appear arbitrary. The two most common procedures for the selection of athletes to be tested is either by lot or on the basis of finishing position. Generally, selection by lot is used in team games (soccer, rugby league, and volleyball) and selection on the basis of finishing position is used in individual sports (triathlon, mountaineering, fencing). Other criteria for identifying athletes for tests include world record breakers (swimming), and those athletes whose behaviour has aroused suspicion (motor sports). The weakness in the testing policy of many federations is most evident in relation to the number of tests conducted with many sports, including ice hockey, taekwondo, yachting and university sports, leaving it to officials at competitions to determine the details of selection for testing. What is particularly interesting to debate is what would be the appropriate criteria for determining whether harmonisation had been achieved with regard to the selection of athletes. Again, uniformity would be inappropriate but the importance of identifying a set of criteria by which sports as diverse as soccer, tennis and motor racing can be judged is a significant challenge and one that the federations seem far from accepting.

One of the most difficult and sensitive aspects of policy harmonisation concerns the sanctions imposed following a doping infraction. As part of the Lausanne Agreement, federations were exhorted to make rapid progress towards the adoption of an agreed set of minimum sanctions for doping infractions, but progress has been extremely slow. Vrijman notes that the IOC established a benchmark for penalties in the late 1980s, suggesting that the penalty for a serious violation of doping rules (anabolic steroids, amphetamines, etc.) should be a ban of two years for a first offence and a life ban for a second offence. For less serious doping infractions involving ephedrine or codeine, for example, the IOC recommended a maximum ban of three months for a first offence, two years for a second and a life ban for a third offence. The strong lead given by the IOC did little to stimulate a consistent approach to sanctions, with a number of federations maintaining lighter penalties and some federations, such as the IAAF in 1991, establishing a harsher penalty of four years for a doping infraction involving drugs such as steroids. The hawkish stance of the IAAF has, however, proved extremely difficult to sustain, with resistance coming from a number of domestic affiliates of the federation and from the legal systems of a small number of major athletic countries, including Germany and the Russian Federation.[1] The difficulty of establishing the initial penalty of four years led the IAAF, in mid 1997, to retreat to a two year initial ban for steroid use. Currently, only the federation responsible for swimming (FINA) is attempting to retain a four year ban. At its recent 1998 meeting in Australia FINA confirmed the four year ban despite being advised by its secretary that it would be vulnerable to challenge in civil courts and in the Court of Arbitration for Sport. To those seeking a more powerful deterrent to drug abuse, the action of the IAAF is seen as a substantial setback but it does force the federation closer to the IOC guidelines of 1988.

On the basis of data available in 1993, Vrijman compared current sanctions with the IOC recommendation and concluded that only twelve of the federations have incorporated the IOC recommended sanctions, while at the same time eleven international sports governing bodies don't seem to apply any sanctions at all! The remaining thirty-one international sports governing bodies have sanctions different from the IOC recommended ones.[2] According to the 1997 survey, the number incorporating the IOC sanctions (or at least very close versions of them) into their rules had risen substantially from twelve to twenty-one which still left the majority of major federations with sets of sanctions that differed from the IOC benchmark or else no sanctions

---

1. Not all legal challenges to the IAAF four year ban have been overturned by national courts. In Britain in 1997 Paul Edwards argued that a four year ban imposed in 1994 for testing positive for steroids should be reduced to two years on the grounds that there were countries where a two year ban was the maximum allowed and the action of the IAAF was consequently discriminatory. The challenge was rejected with the judge concluding that not only was the four year ban reasonable but also that the action of the federation was not discriminatory. *The Times* law report, 30.6.1997.
2. Vrijman, E.N., op. cit., p. 29.

at all! It would be reassuring to establish that the cause of the variation from the IOC standard is due to federations tailoring penalties to suit the particular character and attributes of their sport. To an extent there is evidence to suggest that this is the case. Some federations, such as body building, have harsher penalties, others highlight particular drugs for severe sanctions, such as motor sports with alcohol, and still others have relatively minor variations on the IOC standard. In general, it is a relatively small number of sports that give an impression of neglect or disdain towards the issue. However, the lack of commitment by some federations prompted Juan Antonio Samaranch to raise the issue at the opening of the IOC session prior to the start of the 1998 Nagano winter Olympic Games. He drew attention to the failure of some federations to establish effective out-of-competition testing programmes and appropriately severe sanctions for those guilty of doping infractions.[1]

While it would appear that an increasing number of federations are adopting the IOC set of sanctions, there has been far less progress in persuading federations to recognise the sanctions imposed by other federations. The purpose of such mutual recognition of sanctions is to prevent an athlete banned from participating in one sport simply moving to another sport. In 1993 only five out of fifty-four federations recognised the sanctions imposed by others, and even those five do not recognise the sanctions imposed by government anti-doping agencies, figures that had increased only marginally by 1997.

For those federations that have adopted effective testing regimes and adhere to a set of sanctions it is increasingly important that they also acknowledge the imperatives of natural justice in policy implementation. One central requirement of any set of anti-doping rules is not simply that the analysis of the urine sample is reliable but that the investigation of the allegation of doping be fair, and particularly that the athlete has a right to a hearing. Gay acknowledges that many may conclude that when "the offence of doping is constituted merely by the detection of the presence of a prohibited substance in the urine of an athlete and that prohibited substance has been detected by an accredited laboratory, that there is little point in having a hearing".[2] Gay emphasises that this is a seriously mistaken and dangerous view and argues that "no matter how futile it may seem, every athlete must be given the right, enshrined in the constitution of the governing body, to have the opportunity of a hearing before any final decision is taken as to whether any disciplinary sanctions should be imposed upon that athlete".[3]

Conclusion

Policy harmonisation is never easy to achieve. When harmonisation involves such a wide range of government and private interests the challenge that

---

1. Reuters news report, 2 February 1998.
2. Gay, M. op. cit. p. 5.
3. Ibid., p. 6.

harmonisation presents is formidable indeed. Given that the international anti-doping effort depends so heavily on standardisation of practices and close co-operation between agencies, it is not surprising that harmonisation has emerged in the last ten years as the central priority within the policy area. In that period much has been achieved, particularly as regards the technical aspects of anti-doping procedures. The list of banned substances and practices, the procedures by which samples are collected and analysed, the penalties applied for doping infractions and the basis on which appeals can be made are becoming increasingly comparable across a broad range of Olympic and non-Olympic sports and across a broad range of countries. The effect of this trend has been such that international federations that do not conform to these standards feel obliged to justify their distinctive position.

Growing technical uniformity in anti-doping policy is balanced by a much greater degree of variation in the broader implementation of policy. Agreement on substances to be tested for, the training of sampling officers, and the accreditation of laboratories has proved much easier to achieve than agreement on the number of athletes to be tested, the frequency of testing, and the action to be taken following a positive test result. It is also possible to argue that the progress towards harmonisation has been attained at the expense of the autonomy of sports organisations. It is significant that the strengthening of the international anti-doping policy framework has relied heavily on government action. Over the last ten years, governments have fulfilled a key role in providing the organisational framework, finance and legislative powers for anti-doping initiatives. Anti-doping agencies, established by government and staffed by public officials, with access to public funds to carry out tests and research, and with a legislative basis for their activities are an increasingly common feature of the apparatus of policy implementation.

The growing dominance of public agencies and government departments is the most striking feature of current anti-doping policy. The one possible aspect of policy where sports organisations still retain the initiative is in the establishment of an effective international infrastructure for the development and implementation of policy. While the main governmental forum for policy debate remains the Council of Europe, its effectiveness is limited by the slow pace at which it has been able to promote its Anti-doping Convention beyond Europe. In contrast, the Olympic movement and the major federations, particularly the IAAF, already have a series of well established global forums for policy discussion, such as the IOC and GAISF, as well as the congresses of the individual federations. However, it would be fair to say that the Council of Europe has made far more effective use of its network than either the IOC or the various federation forums.

At this stage in the progress towards greater harmonisation, there is considerable pressure on international sports organisations to recapture the initiative in policy development, with the Lausanne Agreement being an important step in the process. Needless to say, the problems facing both government and sports organisations in implementing an effective anti-doping policy are formidable, not least of which is the long-standing mutual suspicion between the IOC, the federations, and governmental bodies. Other problems include the fragmentation within sport between, for example, commercial and non-commercial sport and between Olympic and non-Olympic sport; the difficulty of establishing criteria by which an acceptable level of harmonisation may be recognised; and the process by which compliance with established standards may be monitored.

Chapter 8

The future of anti-doping policy

Anti-doping policy is at a watershed. It is as though the individuals and organisations involved in the campaign against doping embarked on a sprint only to be told that the race has now become a marathon. Over the last twenty-five years, and especially over the last ten years, there has been substantial progress towards the development of a global anti-doping policy, but each refinement in policy has been accompanied by a sharper insight into the issues and aspects of policy that remain unresolved. There is an unfortunate number of examples of the identification of a problem which prompts a period of enthusiastic debate and policy making, a period which slows considerably when the analysis of the problem leads to a greater awareness of the complexity of the issue or the cost of resources required for its resolution. Initial enthusiasm is dissipated and energy and commitment are sapped creating a situation where, at worst, problems are quietly dropped and attention is given to other more amenable issues.

The initial burst of activity on the issue of doping in sport resulted in a number of important policy developments within a broad range of sports and at major sporting events such as the Olympic Games. Among the most significant developments were the establishment of medical committees across a range of sports, the investment in research to develop testing methods for drugs such as amphetamine, the training of sampling officers, and the effective organisation of drug testing at major sports events. These are all examples of the achievements of the early enthusiasm to deal effectively with drug abuse in sport. As the previous chapter showed, the energy and commitment of the 1980s and 1990s has produced many of the necessary technical requirements for the successful implementation of policy. The widespread acceptance of the IOC list of banned substances and practices, the routine training of sampling officers, the high level of standardisation of sample collection methods, the increasingly routine use of IOC-accredited laboratories for sample analysis, the widespread adoption of the IOC recommended sanctions for doping infractions, are all illustrations of progress in the elaboration of a global anti-doping strategy. The most recent example of the continuing refinement of doping control procedures is the specification of a set of criteria in the form of an ISO 9000 benchmark which should, when finally in place, provide a greater degree of external verification of quality standards in anti-doping policy. More challenging is the constant emergence of new drugs, including those that enhance naturally occurring substances, such as human growth hormones, testosterone, and most recently insulin. Though it is undoubtedly costly to research and develop effective tests for these new substances, the problems are essentially technical and are likely to be resolved given the current level of commitment from governments and some of the larger federations.

Unfortunately, not all the barriers to successful policy implementation are technical. Put starkly, it may well be possible to perfect a series of effective tests for the current crop of new drugs, it may also be possible to establish publicly verifiable quality standards for the sampling and analysis process, and it may be possible to reach a consensus on a scale of penalties for particular doping infractions, but these achievements will count for little if there is not a harmonisation of commitment to tackle the problem of drug abuse by athletes. In other words, alongside the technical questions is a parallel set of questions concerning the values, beliefs and attitudes that are necessary to ensure the maintenance of momentum for implementation. The depth of support for the anti-doping effort among sports organisations and governments is regrettably matched by an equal depth of equivocation and, at times, duplicity among federations and a diminishing, but still significant, number of governments. There is an abundance of evidence that many domestic governing bodies, international federations and governments maintained, during the 1980s in particular, a public commitment to the anti-doping campaign while either simply refusing to enquire too deeply into practices within their own sports or countries or conspiring to subvert the anti-doping strategy of the IOC and the federations.[1] An additional difficulty is that many of the new crop of technical questions, such as blood sampling and liability of the athlete's entourage, are less clear-cut and are complicated by ethical and legal issues that are likely to make their resolution more problematic.

Understanding drug use

It is a truism that policy making should be informed by an understanding, based on research, of the nature of the problem to be addressed. While there has been a considerable investment in researching the problem of drug abuse, it has been skewed heavily in favour of scientific research directed towards the specification of the ergogenic properties of particular drugs and

---

1. See Houlihan, B., *Sport, Policy and Politics*, London, Routledge (1997) for an overview, but see also Australian Government, "Drugs in Sport" interim report of the Senate Standing Committee on the Environment, Recreation and the Arts, Canberra, Australian Government Publishing Service, (1989); Australian Government, "Drugs in Sport" second report of the Senate Standing Committee on the Environment, Recreation and the Arts, Canberra, Australian Government Publishing Service (1989); Dubin Report "Commission of Inquiry into the use of Drugs and Banned Practices Intended to Increase Athletic Performance", Charles Dubin, Commissioner, Ottawa, Canada, Ministry of Supply and Services; Voy, R., *Drugs, Sport and Politics*, Champaign, Ill., Leisure Press (1991); Simson, V. & Jennings, A., *The Lords of the Rings*, London, Simon and Schuster (1992); Jennings, A., *The New Lords of the Rings*, London, Simon & Schuster, (1996).

the development of methods for identifying the presence of prohibited drugs in the athlete's system. This emphasis on the scientific aspects of the problem are understandable but underscores the relative paucity of understanding of the psychological and social aspects of drug use. Thus, although it possible to answer questions with reasonable confidence about the effects of particular drugs on an athlete's performance and the reliability of the tests designed to detect drugs, it is far more difficult to answer the question of why athletes take drugs. Evidence about the motives of athletes is generally anecdotal and offers little beyond the bland assertion that athletes take drugs in order to improve their chances of winning. We know relatively little about how athletes start taking drugs, who introduces them to drugs, how drug use varies by sport, age, gender, or country. We also have at best sparse information about when athletes stop taking drugs, the drug-taking patterns and motivations in non-elite sport and in fringe sporting activities such as body building. Finally, we know little about the level of knowledge among drug abusers about the drugs they take or how they acquire that information.

It would be unfair to suggest that there has been an over-emphasis on the detection and punishment of drug use at the expense of the prevention of the onset of drug use, although it would be fair to argue that it is only comparatively recently that anti-doping agencies have recognised the importance of the provision of information and education as potentially valuable tools in responding to the problem. Over the last five years or so, there has been a much greater investment in the production of information packs and educational material and there has also been a shift in emphasis in this material, away from reliance on appeals to the sense of fair play of athletes and to an emphasis on providing information about the serious health risks associated with drug abuse. One of the best examples of increasing sophistication in the understanding of the social context of drug use is the research carried out by the Australian Sports Drug Agency (ASDA). ASDA has conducted a series of surveys of athletes and of coaches designed to gather data, for example, about the level of knowledge about drugs, the perceived effectiveness of the current anti-doping programme, the extent to which coaches are involved in anti-doping activity, and where athletes and coaches obtain their information about drugs. On the basis of this data, ASDA has been able to refine and target more precisely its educational programme.

It is becoming increasingly apparent that education and the provision of information are likely to remain key elements of the anti-doping strategy and a necessary complement to the longer established policy of deterrence through detection and punishment. However, if education is to be an effective tool in the anti-doping strategy then it needs to be informed by a more comprehensive understanding of the context of drug use in sport. In addition, it is important to bear in mind the need to identify the appropriate targets for information and education. While few would deny that the athlete and the aspiring athlete are primary targets, with coaches, sports doctors and sports administrators a set of secondary targets, it is important not to ignore the need to keep the general public informed and educated about drug use in sport. It would be of little value to create a situation where drug using athletes were a pariah group among other athletes if they were still treated as heroes and heroines by sponsors, the press and the public.

The threat of legal challenge

Distasteful as many involved in sport may find it, sport and the law are intimately intertwined. Nowhere is the interconnection between sport and law more evident than in relation to doping. In general, the courts in many countries have been disinclined to intervene in matters concerning the organisation and conduct of sport whether it involves matters of eligibility or athlete behaviour. Nevertheless, the courts have steadily (even if reluctantly) extended their involvement with sport. In part this is the result of a broader trend in many countries to seek redress through the courts as a first course of action rather than as a last resort, but it is also the result of the rapid commercialisation of sport and the fact that there are an increasing number of athletes who stand to lose substantial earnings if their careers are interrupted through suspension. Added to these reasons is the reluctance among commercial clubs and businesses, such as television companies, to lose star players due to positive drug tests. In the previous chapter, mention was made of the recent spate of high profile challenges to the decisions of anti-doping agencies and domestic and international federations. What is striking about recent cases is not just the number of them but the variety of bases on which legal challenges are being mounted. First, there are those, like Martin Vinnicombe, who are admitted drug takers and who avoid sanctions due to inconsistencies between the regulations of the anti-doping agencies. Second, there are those, like Katrin Krabbe, who mount successful challenges to the scale of penalty applied for the doping infraction. Thirdly, there are those, such as Diane Modahl, who having established their innocence, have then used the courts to seek damages against the responsible sports organisation.[1] Finally, there are a large number of potential legal challenges from athletes penalised for doping infractions in the early years of the anti-doping campaign for whom the current crop of challenges provide a powerful demonstration of the possible grounds for disputing earlier decisions. For example, it was reported recently that the American swimmer, Rick DeMont, is attempting to sue the United States Olympic Committee for US$ 12 million in connection with its decision in 1972 to strip him of his Olympic gold medal following a

---

1. It is interesting to note that the IAAF expects national governing bodies to deal with the hearing and all the related expenses, but reserves the right to arbitrate in a decision of the national federation. The settlement of Diane Modahl's claim is complicated by the recent bankruptcy of the British Athletics Federation which was partly the result of the costs associated with the Modahl case.

positive test for ephedrine, a drug contained in an asthma treatment he was using at the time.[1]

To these well-publicised cases that have reached, or are likely to reach, the courts must be added the large number of cases in which findings have been overturned by sports arbitration panels or tribunals. In 1994, in the United Kingdom, seven cases had been overturned or shelved by governing bodies often due to a rejection of, or lack of confidence in, laboratory results. In the same year there had also been two cases in Austria, including one where an athlete sued the international federation for loss of earnings because it had applied a four year ban, one year longer than the domestic governing body. Similar cases, where sanctions had not been applied for doping infractions, were reported from the Netherlands, where cases have been dropped because the testosterone/epitestosterone ratios were considered borderline, and from Norway, where a positive result was not deemed to be a doping infraction because of a lack of "intent" on the part of the athlete and a lack of proven effect of the drug. It is not just the growing number of appeals against the decisions in doping cases that is notable but also the variety of grounds on which appeals are based, both factors which reinforce the need for clearly and precisely worded anti-doping regulations and for adherence to a set of rigorous standards covering the sampling and analytical processes. The increasing prevalence of legal challenges to test results and the decisions of anti-doping authorities provide a powerful imperative for greater harmonisation among federations and national anti-doping agencies. Greater harmonisation should reduce the opportunities for successful legal challenges arising from inconsistency between the rules of different agencies. In addition, the process of harmonisation should enable a diffusion of best practice and the consequent reduction in appeals that exploit the inadequacies of federation rule books.

Blood sampling

It is clearly apparent that the need to take account of the vulnerability to appeal is a theme that runs through any discussion of present anti-doping policy and any proposals for change. The current discussion of the introduction of blood sampling is a case in point. Blood sampling offers the prospect of, first, greater accuracy in analysis, second, an opportunity to provide corroboration for the results of urine analysis, and third, the opportunity to test for a wider range of drugs and banned practices. Blood sampling is a far more promising way of identifying the use of the newer generation of drugs, especially those related to rEPO and growth hormones. Indeed the research project GH2000, jointly funded by the IOC and the European Union and aimed at detecting the use of growth hormone preparations by athletes, is based on the use of blood samples. In addition, the use of blood sampling is also a pos-

---

1. Reported in *The Times* (London), 28 July 1997.

sible way of combating manipulation of testosterone/epitestosterone ratios through the establishment of a database of individual testosterone/epitestosterone ratios so as to recognise, more accurately, aberrant ratios. Although the Council of Europe recognises the potential value of blood testing in identifying heterologous blood doping, it has been reluctant to promote its use because of the relative lack of scientific confirmation of its utility in identifying homologous blood doping and the presence of drugs such as rEPO and other peptide hormones. Nevertheless, the Monitoring Group of the Anti-doping Convention has been investigating the ethical and legal aspects of blood sampling for the last three years and has prepared a draft set of guidelines on blood sampling, should the IOC or the federations decide to adopt blood sampling as a major doping control method.

Blood sampling has been used on a limited and experimental basis by a number of federations including the IAAF which, in 1993, carried out forty-eight tests over four competitions, largely as a way of identifying the issues that would need to be addressed if blood sampling were to become more extensive. The International Ski Federation introduced testing in 1989 at the Nordic World Ski Championships and was given permission by the IOC to undertake fifty-five blood tests at the Lillehammer winter Olympics in 1994. More interestingly, cycling has, for a number of years, operated a system of "blood control" which involves the removal of a small blood sample (by pricking the athlete's finger) and testing for a very limited number of forms of blood manipulation through measurement of the haemoglobin and haematocrit levels. If these levels are significantly elevated the rider is informed that his/her blood is not in a suitable condition for competition and he or she is "banned" for fifteen days.[1] The ban is seen as a way of safeguarding the health of the rider. Despite the ambiguity of the interpretation of the results of the analysis of the blood sample, the impact has been to reduce substantially the number of riders with unusually high readings.[2]

If the focus for doping control analysis is to shift from urine to blood, it would appear that just at the time when the sports community is tackling the issue of harmonisation of doping control based on urine analysis there is a risk that momentum will be lost by the introduction of a whole series of new issues surrounding the use of blood. In a report prepared by Bahr et al on behalf of the Lillehammer Olympic Organising Committee, the differences between doping control based on urine analysis and that based on blood sampling were highlighted and included the following: blood sampling is new to

---

1. In May 1997 the Italian cyclist, Claudio Chiappucci, failed a blood test during a competition and was suspended for fifteen days. His red blood cell level was 51%, just over the limit of 50%. Chiappucci was the fourth rider to have failed a blood test since the regulations were introduced.
2. One outcome of the current series of investigations by the French police into the use of EPO during the 1998 Tour de France are claims that the blood tests are not effective in detecting those who might have used the drug because riders are given 90 minutes notice of a test, which is sufficient time to dilute the blood and lower the haematocrit level.

athletes; it is invasive and may cause anxiety and pain; blood is not a waste product and affects the oxygen-carrying capacity of the body; on-site preparation of blood samples may be required; blood sampling carries a slight risk of infection; venepuncture would require trained medical staff; and there is the increased risk of disease infection.

Blood sampling is new to nearly all athletes and would therefore require the kind of information and education campaign that has been mounted by many countries and sports to promote urine analysis. In addition, there may be problems in securing the political, legal and cultural acceptance of blood sampling within certain countries. At present, with blood sampling being, for most sports, at the discussion stage, there are few specific problems of acceptance. However, it must be stressed that there has been, as yet, no test in the courts of the legality of blood sampling and there is the example of Austria where blood testing for non-medical purposes is unlawful. There is also a wider concern that blood testing as a requirement might be in breach of both the European Convention on Human Rights and the Convention on Human Rights and Biomedicine.

The range of potential legal implications of blood sampling is broad and daunting and includes the question of liability for injury received or illness contracted as a result of blood collection. In addition, there would need to be clarification of the implications of customs regulations for the transport of blood across borders. Further clarification would be required concerning the implications of domestic public health laws, for example concerning any requirement to provide information on infectious diseases identified during analysis for drugs. Caution in allowing blood sampling is understandable and in part reflects a legal concern with liability and also a desire to protect the individual from unnecessary anxiety and pain. For a minority, antipathy towards blood sampling reflects a more deep-rooted ethical objection to interfering with the human body. Following a survey by the IOC in 1991 it would appear that the only major religious group that would find blood sampling unacceptable is the Jehovah's Witnesses.

While the collection of urine samples might be embarrassing for athletes, it is not an invasive technique. In contrast, blood testing would be invasive and would require the collection of a substantial sample of around twenty cubic centimetres. Although there is a concern that blood is not a waste product like urine, and that blood also fulfils an important function in maximising energy efficiency in the athlete through its function in transporting oxygen, it is also recognised that a sample of twenty cubic centimetres will not affect the body's efficiency and that the quantity removed is replaced within twelve hours.

Depending on the type of tests to be undertaken, blood may need to be separated, by means of clotting, or centrifugation, for example, into its distinct components, such as plasma, serum and red blood cells, prior to analysis.

Depending on the tests to be carried out, some processes may need to be completed before the blood or its constituents can be transported to the laboratory. The most obvious implication of on-site preparation of blood samples is the increase in cost that is implied. Escalation in cost may also be due to the likely requirement that medically qualified staff would have to be employed to collect samples through venepuncture and also because handling blood necessitates a higher level of skill and care due to the increased risk of infection. However, while the greater risk of infection for staff handling blood samples requires higher levels of technical skill, the analysis of samples also raises at least two important ethical issues. The first issue concerns the ethics of the suggestion that the blood samples would be an important resource for wider medical research and that once the drugs tests had been undertaken the samples should be made available for general medical research. Second, there is the more important ethical question regarding the notification of diseases, such as anaemia or HIV-disease, to athletes (and possibly to health authorities in some countries) identified incidentally during the analysis for drugs.

Despite these specific issues associated with the wide scale introduction of blood testing in sport, there is a view in the monitoring group that the Council's existing recommendation on standard urine procedures could be applied, *mutatis mutandis*, to a new recommendation on blood. Moreover, a frequently expressed view by the supporters of blood testing is that blood sampling is an increasingly common feature in sports training and in everyday life. For example, most countries routinely use the collection and analysis of blood samples as part of the tests for alcohol in the blood stream of motor vehicle drivers. Indeed, one respondent to the IOC survey of opinion argued that many athletes routinely have their blood analysed as part of the monitoring of their health and as part of the assessment of training effectiveness through the monitoring of lactate levels. In addition, the point was made that blood sampling was less intrusive and less demeaning than the taking of a urine sample, and also quicker, as the delay in obtaining a urine sample from dehydrated athletes would be avoided.

Despite the growing evidence that blood sampling will provide a more secure and effective basis on which to identify doping infractions, it is likely that for the foreseeable future blood sampling will fulfil a supplementary role to current urine tests. This situation is the result of the problems mentioned above connected with the technical and especially the financial implications of the widespread adoption of blood sampling, but is also an acknowledgement of the need to establish the legal and cultural acceptability of blood sampling, the minimisation of the associated medical risks, and the basis on which consent to provide a blood sample can be assumed. Emile Vrijman of the Netherlands Centre for Doping Affairs argued recently for a reduction in the momentum for the introduction of blood testing until it could be established more clearly that the advantages of the method outweighed the additional cost and difficulties in replacing the well established system of doping control based on urine analysis.[1]

One issue at the heart of progress towards harmonisation, especially if this includes blood doping, is the definition of the relationship between the athlete and his/her domestic governing body and international federation. During the years when the title "amateur" had some significance, the model of the relationship was one which viewed sportsmen and women as members of a club with the obligations that membership carried. More recently, as commercialisation of sport has led to emergence across a broader range of sports of the professional athlete, the analogy of the "club" and of "membership" has been replaced by one which talks of "business" and "employees". Within the IOC there is an acknowledgement that the relationship between athletes and their federation is increasingly being subsumed under employment and contract law, hence a growing support within the committee for the notion that athletes should be regarded as employees with obligations as well as rights. The relevance of this potential development is that it is increasingly common for employers to insist on periodic drug tests of their employees, most obviously in transport and security industries but also in some office-based industries. In countries, such as Australia, where drug testing in sport is supported by specific legislation, the shifting definition of the athlete-federation relationship and the growth of workplace testing will merely provide additional reinforcement of the acceptance of testing. Whether drug testing in sport is based on dedicated legislation or not, the trend to viewing athletes as comparable to other employees is likely to complicate progress towards harmonisation. On the one hand, employment law in many countries, with its heavy emphasis on the obligation of the employee to have regard for the safety of others in the course of his/her duties, will reinforce many of the objectives of the advocates of harmonisation. On the other hand, there is a danger that in those countries where drug testing in sport is dependent on convention and agreement, any move to extend the remit of employment law to sport may make harmonisation more difficult to achieve.

Harmonisation of sanctions

One of the issues that appears to be increasingly intractable is the harmonisation of sanctions. There are two related aspects to the problem. First, attempts to treat all sports in the same way and second, the division of drugs into two or at most three very broad categories. Their concern is that sanctions should be more sensitive to the particular characteristics of the sport, especially the typical length of a career, and also sensitive to the differential benefit of the same drug in different sports. Within most legal systems, punishment is a mix of mandatory penalties (usually for the minor crimes, such as motoring

1. Vrijman, E. N., *Blood Sampling and Doping Control*, Netherlands Centre for Doping Affairs (1995).

offences, and for the most serious crimes, such as murder) and penalties which can be imposed at the discretion of the judge, but usually within legislative guidelines. With regard to doping there are some sports, such as cycling and athletics, that have developed a bespoke set of penalties, but generally federations adopt the IOC recommended tariff of sanctions. For some federations the willingness to adopt the IOC tariff is a mark of apathy rather than commitment, but for others it reflects an acknowledgement of risks associated with applying penalties to athletes and the security to be gained from applying a penalty that has a legitimacy based on common action with the IOC and other major federations. At this relatively early stage in policy development, it is important that the IOC and the federations establish a set of guideline sanctions that are effective in deterring drug users and which command sufficient respect among athletes and federations to act as a reference point for debates within individual sports about the refinement of sanctions to meet the precise characteristics of their sport. To this end, and following considerable debate among sports organisations, the IOC developed such a set of reference sanctions, with a two year ban for a first offence involving steroids being a key aspect. As mentioned in the previous chapter, the IAAF, in particular, but also the International Weightlifting Federation and FINA wished to adopt or retain a stronger sanction for a first offence involving steroids. The recent decision by the IAAF to retreat from its policy may be seen as a welcome reinforcement of the IOC lead, but this would be a rationalisation of policy weakness on the part of the IAAF.

The status of the IAAF as the major Olympic sports federation, and ranking alongside federations such as FIFA among Olympic and non-Olympic federations, gives its actions a particular significance. It has already been mentioned that the second stage of policy development regarding sanctions would be for individual sports to shape sanctions to suit their distinctive characteristics. Only a small number of federations, such as those for cycling, weightlifting and athletics, have taken that step. The decision of the IAAF to bring its penalties closer to those of the IOC is likely to undermine the modest momentum towards refinement of sanctions that was emerging. It will consequently become much more difficult for other federations to sustain the imposition of sanctions that exceed the IOC guidelines and will also deter those federations that were considering any deviation from the IOC model. More worrying is the basis on which the IAAF retreat was made, namely the defeat in the courts in one member state. The key decision was that made by the Munich Regional Appeal Court in March 1995 which declared that Katrin Krabbe's suspension for a three year period for steroid use was invalid because a suspension of "more than two years contravenes (...) the constitutional principle of proportionality".[1] The decision of the German court came at about the same time that the British courts were rejecting the appeal by Paul Edwards against a

---

similar IAAF-imposed four year ban and the Canadian court was rejecting Ben Johnson's appeal against his life ban. If progress towards harmonisation on sanctions is to be dictated by the particularities of the legal system in one country, then harmonisation will only be possible if it based on the acceptance of the "lowest common denominator". The policy of harmonisation consequently runs the risk of becoming a rationalisation of failure.

The jurisdiction of anti-doping bodies

A further crucial aspect of current policy which needs clarification if progress to greater harmonisation is to be maintained concerns the management of the overlapping jurisdictions of the various organisations involved in anti-doping. Given the widespread public condemnation of doping by sports bodies and governments, it is surprising the speed with which organisations will protest at what they perceive to be an invasion of their jurisdiction. The view of UEFA is not uncommon. Not only has UEFA argued that it is not able to undertake out-of-competition testing because the workload is too great, but it has also objected to national doping agencies carrying out tests at UEFA competitions. The problem of overlapping jurisdictions is the product of the fragmented evolution of anti-doping policies in different countries and sports. Clashes of jurisdiction are unlikely to occur during major international competitions, such as the Olympic Games, when there is a long-established precedent of testing by the organising body. Jurisdictional friction is more likely where a competition takes place over a long period of time, such as a cricket test match series or a soccer competition where there is a clear need for agreement between the domestic doping agency and the international federation about jurisdiction. Conflict is even more likely in the case of out-of-competition testing by international federations which may take place without the national anti-doping authority being informed.

Leaving aside the territorial concerns of the various agencies, the range of testing bodies is confusing for athletes who may be tested by officers of their international federation, by the officers of the anti-doping agency of the country in which they are currently located, and by officers of the organising body of the competition in which they participate. Superficially the problem of overlapping jurisdiction can be easily solved through a combination of greater courtesy by agencies in informing others of their intentions and actions and the fostering of a higher level of mutual confidence. At a more fundamental level, the prescription for the resolution of the problem may be far less easy to achieve. Raising the level of mutual confidence is likely to be especially problematic. Greater mutual confidence is required not just in the capacity of agencies to undertake drug testing effectively, but also in the motives of other agencies. For the federations, the maintenance of jurisdictional boundaries reflects a deeper concern to prevent an erosion of control over their sport and taps a deeply held suspicion of the long-term commitment of governments to sport. Developing a degree of mutual confidence sufficient to encourage federations to cede authority to national doping agencies is a long-term project and one that must provide federations (and not just the sport for which they are responsible) with a tangible benefit.

The athlete's entourage

Just at the time when the harmonisation of primary aspects of anti-doping policy such as sanctions and jurisdiction are becoming more problematic, other issues, including the punishment of members of the athlete's entourage for involvement in doping, are being added to the harmonisation agenda. In 1994, it was agreed by members of the Council of Europe's monitoring group to raise the profile of the issue of the role of an athlete's entourage in doping. The Anti-doping Convention refers to the importance of encouraging sports organisations to harmonise their "procedures for the imposition of effective penalties for officials, doctors, veterinary doctors, coaches, physiotherapists and other officials or accessories associated with infringements of the anti-doping regulations by sportsmen and women".[1] Over recent years this aspect of the convention has grown in importance particularly as a result of the steady reduction in the age of elite athletes in many sports such as gymnastics, swimming, skating and tennis and the occurrence of positive drug tests among minors. The concern with the behaviour of the athlete's entourage in relation to doping is thus reinforced by the increasing concern to curtail incidents of abuse of young athletes through, for example, manipulation of diet and over-training. However, the problems involved in punishing an athlete's entourage are substantial even when the athlete is a minor. The current anti-doping policy is focused on the athlete and there has been little discussion, let alone experience, of establishing a procedure for examining the involvement of others.[2] In addition, as part of the drive for greater harmonisation, federations are being encouraged to define doping purely in terms of strict liability, a concept that is difficult to apply to the athlete's entourage, with the possible though arguable exception of those associated with athletes who are minors. Also, athletes accused of a doping infraction have a right to a hearing which is investigative and clarificatory in nature: any hearings involving others would, of necessity, be adversarial in nature. Finally, and of overwhelming importance, is the stark fact that federations barely have the resources to support anti-doping programmes aimed at athletes and are unlikely to be able to produce the additional resources that an extension of the policy would require. As a result the recommendation published by the Council of Europe regarding the involvement of an athlete's entourage in doping is an example of policy as aspiration rather than as substance.[3]

---

1. Council of Europe Anti-doping Convention, Article 7.2e (1989).
2. Cycling and swimming are two exceptions.
3. A further source of concern is the apparent willingness of countries to employ coaches from the former GDR. Australia has recently appointed Ekkart Arbeit as its head coach despite the fact that Arbeit is under investigation for his involvement in government-sanctioned doping. According to Werner Franke, the German parliamentary investigator, Arbeit was "a major person responsible for the use of anabolic steroids" (The *Guardian* newspaper, 3.10.1997). However, Germany employs the former East German swimming coach, Winfried Leopold, despite his admission that he was involved in doping in the 1980s.

One suggestion that emerged during the discussion of the ways in which young athletes could be protected from doping and other forms of exploitation was to place a heavier responsibility on the domestic governing body to safeguard actively the interests of children. The notion that domestic governing bodies should take greater responsibility for the actions of their athletes and officials is one that is gaining some support as a strategy in the campaign against doping. The threat by FINA to suspend domestic governing bodies whose athletes had an especially poor record of drug offences was partly responsible for the greater openness in China about its recent drug record. This followed a similar policy adopted by the International Weightlifting Federation. Such strategies for encouraging compliance by domestic governing bodies can be effective but depend obviously on the commitment of the international federation to opposing doping. A source of pressure on international federations comes from the governing bodies in countries where there exists a government-resourced anti-doping policy or where there has been a tradition of success in the particular sport which is being threatened by weaker anti-doping policies in other countries. Canada would be a good example of the former and the United States an example of the latter. The United States' governing body for swimming strongly supported the proposed suspension of the Chinese from international competition for two reasons: first, it strongly suspected the Chinese governing body of either actively or passively supporting drug abuse by its swimmers; and, second, because the rapid success of the Chinese swimmers was challenging the traditional American dominance resulting in fewer Olympic medals and consequently a smaller share of USOC finance.

The future of anti-doping policy

The substantial progress that has been made over the last ten years or so in refining anti-doping policy and its implementation has to be balanced against the emergence of a series of new issues (including blood sampling) and new aspects of longer-established issues (jurisdictional friction, retreat on sanctions, and doping and minors). It would not be over-dramatising the current state of policy to suggest that anti-doping policy is at a crucial stage in its evolution. One way of conceptualising the challenge facing anti-doping authorities is to view progress on anti-doping as a linear progression along the upward curve of a graph. According to this model, the goal is both clear and within sight but each succeeding move towards the goal is more difficult to achieve. However, progress is sustained by a consensus among interested parties over the policy goal and also over the means by which it is to be attained. Although accurate in indicating the progressive difficulty in making headway, an alternative model is one which is three-dimensional rather than linear, which is stepped rather than represented by a smooth curve and where the goal is occasionally clear but at other times lost in a fog of re-negotiation. The three-dimensional aspect takes account of the continuing debates about the best means of achieving anti-doping objectives and would include debates over complementing urine tests with blood sampling, the proper balance between in-competition, and out-of-competition tests, and the respective roles and jurisdictions of national anti-doping agencies, the IOC and the federations. The periodic indistinctness of policy goals represents the admittedly occasional disagreements over whether to include particular drugs, test particular groups of athletes and extend the remit beyond elite competitive sport. The steps are by far the most important element in the model as they represent a quantum break or watershed in policy development where continued progress is no longer possible given the current level of resources. The late 1980s was one such watershed, and occurred when the limitations of in-competition testing had become all too apparent and the extension of out-of-competition testing required considerable additional, and qualitatively different, resources such as authority, money and technical expertise. The current watershed is rather less focused than that of the late 1980s and includes the delay, and continuing problems, in developing reliable tests for some of the hormone-based drugs, the rising cost of research programmes aimed at identifying tests for new drugs, the likely escalation in the cost of conducting tests should blood sampling be more widely adopted, and the sensitivity among federations that their role in anti-doping is being usurped by governmental agencies.[1] Central to all these elements of current policy is the concern that the necessary organisational commitment from governments, the IOC and the federations to achieve the quantum change in policy is lacking.

There is substantial evidence of a lack of political will among some governments and sports bodies underlying their public protestations of support for drug-free sport. Allegations persist of unreported positives on the one hand and, on the other, reported positives where no action was taken at recent Olympic Games. Many commentators have detected a lack of enthusiasm among senior members of the IOC for an intensive anti-doping programme. A similar impression of muted enthusiasm is formed when assessing the commitment of the federations. Federations have to cope with increasingly assertive athletes and clubs, and, globally, are under intense pressure to retain their authority and control over major events and competitions. Some federations, such as those for rugby (both union and league) and soccer, are definitely the weaker partner in the relationship, with elite clubs mirroring the erosion of federation power that has already taken place in golf, tennis and some motor sports.

---

1. One cost which is of growing concern relates to the maintenance of IOC-accredited laboratories. There are seventeen accredited labs in Europe but many of the smaller ones are finding it difficult to survive. Laboratories are estimated to need between 10 000 and 30 000 samples for analysis each year in order to be economically viable. As a result there might only be scope for five or six laboratories in Europe. In addition, there is the increasing cost of laboratory equipment and staff. For example, a high resolution mass spectrometer costs approximately US$ 600 000, is expensive to run and needs highly qualified (and well paid) staff to operate it.

It would be of some comfort to be able to demonstrate that governments still evince a higher level of collective probity regarding doping, but while a number have taken a lead in providing the political and tangible resources required to maintain the momentum of anti-doping policy, there is also a number whose failure to reinforce their rhetoric with action arouses and sustains suspicion regarding their intentions. The expectation that government-supported doping had ended with the fall of communism has proved to be over-optimistic.

It is within this context of pressing technical and scientific problems and variable political and organisational support that efforts towards greater harmonisation are taking place. Despite the challenging context for harmonisation, there are a number of positive developments which augur well for the future. Most notable is the number of examples of co-operation on anti-doping issues between government and sports organisations. At the scientific level, the GH2000 project aimed at developing a test to identify the presence of growth hormones relies on joint funding of £1.8 million by the IOC and the European Union. As mentioned earlier, the European Union was also involved in the joint production of *The Clean Sport Guide* along with the Council of Europe. The 1994 Lausanne Agreement is a further example of co-operation between sports organisations being supported by all the key organisations within the Olympic movement, including the associations of both summer and winter Olympic federations (ASOIF & AIWF), the International Olympic Federations, the Association of National Olympic Committees and the various continental associations of NOCs. More importantly, the IOC-sponsored working group (Harmonisation of Rules on Doping Control) inspired by the Lausanne Agreement draws its membership from federations, national governmental doping control agencies, and from the Council of Europe.

The above examples provide illustrations of the extent to which an inter-organisational infrastructure is emerging which enables contact and discussions between the different interests. It also draws attention to the number of different clusters of interests that need to be involved in the harmonisation process. Harmonisation involves at least two parallel processes, the first within the various clusters and the second between clusters. Among the clusters of interests that may be readily identified are the international federations, governments, and the IOC. The first process focuses on the harmonisation of policy within individual sports between domestic governing bodies and the parent federation, among federations and among governments, while the second process involves the harmonisation between governmental and non-governmental sports organisations. Even with three major clusters the problems of harmonisation would be formidable, but in reality each cluster can be further divided into subsets of interests. For example, the federations may be divided between the Olympic and non-Olympic, the rich and poor, the established and the new, and those that are commercially successful and those that are not. Each main cluster is, at best, a loose and sometimes uneasy coalition of interests all generally capable of withholding their support from proposals of which they are suspicious. One could be forgiven for asking whether the harmonisation project is over-ambitious, as the issue is too complex and there are just too many organisations with a capacity to prevaricate and veto policy. However, rather than this line of questioning leading to a concern about the prospects for policy success, it should prompt a reflection on the importance of establishing criteria against which progress towards harmonisation may be measured and also a set of broad agreements about the extent of harmonisation that would constitute successful policy implementation.

Harmonisation, as an outcome, is far from easy to define and has at least two important dimensions that need to be taken into account: namely, depth and breadth. Depth, in relation to doping, has three elements: first, the extent of change required in national policies; second, the degree to which states and other bodies, such as federations, have to adopt policies that they would not otherwise adopt; and third, the extent to which policy prescription extends beyond general statements of values and addresses matters of operational detail. The progress that has been made in encouraging governments to formulate explicit policies towards doping and the decline in the number of governments seeking to subvert the anti-doping campaign indicates substantial success in terms of the first element. The second element is more problematic, with the United States in particular having considerable difficulty in establishing an effective anti-doping regime in a political and legal system which is so strongly committed to protecting the rights of the individual. There is considerable evidence that policy has depth when measured in terms of an emphasis on the detail with which it expressed. This is particularly the case with regard to matters associated with urine sample collection, transport and analysis, but increasingly the case in relation to the procedures to be adopted in any disciplinary hearing and subsequent appeal.

Harmonisation can also be assessed in terms of breadth, which refers to the proportion of potential parties to an agreement to harmonise that is deemed to be sufficient for satisfactory compliance.[1] What is the critical mass required in order to maintain the commitment of the supporters of harmonisation? Taking the 190-plus members of the Olympic movement, it might be possible to argue that, as long as the thirty or so most successful medal-winning countries comply, there will be little concern about failures of compliance by the others. A much more serious question is the extent of non-compliance by strong Olympic countries needed to undermine progress towards harmonisation. The non-compliance of the former GDR and Soviet Union clearly weakened western commitment to anti-doping. This aspect of breadth is

---

1. See Chayes, A. & Chayes, A.H., "On compliance", *International Organisation*, 47, pp. 175-205, 1993.

important especially in relation to the large number of states whose capacity to comply is determined as much by availability of resources as by political commitment to anti-doping objectives.

Assuming that measures of depth and breadth could be specified with sufficient precision, implementation of policy and the monitoring of compliance on a global level is daunting and potentially extremely expensive. It is possibly for this reason that there has been a trend in recent years towards a series of regional or small-scale attempts at harmonisation. The Nordic Anti-doping Agreement and the signatories of the International Anti-Doping Agreement, plus the growing number of bilateral agreements, are all making important contributions towards greater harmonisation, and the danger of fragmentation of effort is outweighed by the value of being able to identify examples of effective harmonisation which may then act as examples of good practice for other governments and sports organisations to follow. In reality, the fostering of global forums for policy discussion complemented by more regional or localised experiments in harmonisation of policy implementation is likely to prove the most effective strategy for maintaining policy momentum over the coming years.

Yet the key requirement for sustained policy momentum is the continued provision of scientific, organisational and political support from a range of key organisations and groups including governments, the major federations and the Olympic movement. Of these ingredients for continued policy momentum, the most important is a high level of broadly based political support, not just from governments but, probably more importantly, from the public. Possibly the greatest threat to the anti-doping campaign is that the public loses interest in the issue. As was made clear in Chapter 5, arguments to underpin the anti-doping policy based on notions of fairness, health, paternalism and role model behaviour are too vulnerable to charges of inconsistency to provide a sufficient justification for the present policy. The foundation of existing policy and the determining factors in assuring closer harmonisation are sustained disapproval of doping by the majority of those involved in sport and the continuing vocal public support for current anti-doping efforts.

Possibly the greatest danger at the present time is that the debate on the future direction of policy becomes too esoteric for the public, too much the province of experts, and too disassociated from the sports that the mass of the public play and events that the public enjoy watching. The current attention being paid to the array of legal, technical and scientific issues generated by the harmonisation debate is a necessary step in policy refinement, but it is also important not to lose sight of the importance of keeping the public educated about the issues in order to ensure continued support. The Modahl, Krabbe and Vinnicombe cases are all in their various ways policy failures that give added urgency to the drive for closer harmonisation. These cases have the effect of, at best, confusing the public and, at worst, sowing the seeds of cynicism so evident in public attitudes to drug abuse by American football players and which results in each new positive result producing a shrug of the shoulders rather than an emphatic condemnation.

Appendices

Appendix A

International Olympic Committee list of prohibited classes of substances and prohibited methods

31 January 1998

I.   Prohibited classes of substances

A. Stimulants
B. Narcotics
C. Anabolic Agents
D. Diuretics
E. Peptide and glycoprotein hormones and analogues

II.   Prohibited methods

A. Blood doping
B. Pharmacological, chemical and physical manipulation

III. Classes of drugs subject to certain restrictions

A. Alcohol
B. Marijuana
C. Local anaesthetics
D. Corticosteroids
E. Beta-blockers

I.   Prohibited classes of substances

Prohibited substances fall into the following classes of substances:

A.   Stimulants
B.   Narcotics
C.   Anabolic Agents
D.   Diuretics
E.   Peptide and glycoprotein hormones and analogues

All substances belonging to the prohibited classes cannot be used even if they are not listed as examples. For this reason, the term "and related substances" is introduced. This term describes drugs that are related to the class by their pharmacological action and/or chemical structure.

A. *Stimulants*

Prohibited substances in class A include the following examples:

amineptine, amiphenazole, amphetamines, bromantan, caffeine*, carphedon, cocaine, ephedrines**, fencamfamine, mesocarb, pentylentetrazol, pipradol, salbutamol***, salmeterol***, terbutaline***, and related substances.

* For caffeine the definition of a positive result depends on the concentration of caffeine in the urine. The concentration in urine may not exceed 12 micrograms per millilitre.

** For ephedrine, cathine and methylephedrine, the definition of a positive is 5 micrograms per millilitre of urine. For phenylpropanolamine and pseudoephedrine the definition of a positive is 10 micrograms per millilitre. If more than one of these substances is present, the quantities should be added, and, if the sum exceeds 10 micrograms per millilitre the sample shall be considered positive.

*** Permitted by inhaler only when their use is previously certified in writing by a respiratory or team physician to the relevant medical authority.

Note: All imidazole preparations are acceptable for topical use, e.g. oxymetazoline. Vasoconstrictors (e.g. adrenaline) may be administered with local anaesthetic agents. Topical preparations (e.g. nasal, ophthalmological) of phenylephrine are permitted.

B. *Narcotics*

Prohibited substances in class B include the following examples:

dextromoramide, diamorphine (heroin), methadone, morphine, pentazocine, pethidine

and related substances.

Note: codeine, dextromethorphan, dextropropoxyphene, dihydrocodeine, diphenoxylate, ethylmorphine, pholcodine and propoxyphene are permitted.

C. *Anabolic agents*

The Anabolic class includes: 1. anabolic androgenic steroids (AAS) and 2. beta-2 agonists.

Prohibited substances in class C include the following examples:

1. *Anabolic androgenic steroids*

androstenedione, clostebol, dehydroepiandrosterone (DHEA), fluoxymesterone, metandienone, metenolone, nandrolone, oxandrolone, stanozolol, testosterone*, and related substances.

* The presence of a testosterone (T) to epitestosterone (E) ratio greater than six to one in the urine of a competitor constitutes an offence unless there is evidence that this ratio is due to a physiological or pathological condition, e.g. low epitestosterone excretion, androgen-producing tumour, enzyme deficiencies.

In the case of T/E higher than six, it is mandatory that the relevant medical authority conduct an investigation before the sample is declared positive. A full report will be written and will include a review of previous tests, subsequent tests and any results of endocrine investigations. In the event that previous tests are not available, the athlete should be tested unannounced at least once per month for three months. The results of these investigations should be included in the report. Failure to co-operate in the investigations will result in declaring the sample positive.

2. Beta-2 agonists

When administered systemically, beta-2 agonists may have powerful anabolic effects.

Clenbuterol, fenoterol, salbutamol, salmeterol, terbutaline and related substances.

D. Diuretics

Prohibited substances in class D include the following examples:

acetazolamide, bumetanide, chlorthalidone, ethacrynic acid, furosemide, hydrochlorothiazide, mannitol*, mersalyl, spironolactone, triamterene, and related substances.

* Prohibited by intravenous injection.

E. Peptide and glycoprotein hormones and analogues

Prohibited substances in class E include the following examples:

1. Chorionic Gonadotrophin (hCG – human chorionic gonadotrophin);
2. Corticotrophin (ACTH);
3. Growth hormone (hGH – somatotrophin);

All the respective releasing factors (and their analogues) of the above-mentioned substances are also prohibited.

4. Erythropoietin (EPO)

II. Prohibited methods

The following procedures are prohibited:

A. *Blood doping*

Blood doping is the administration of blood, red blood cells and related blood products to an athlete. This procedure may be preceded by withdrawal of blood from the athlete who continues to train in this blood depleted state.

B. *Pharmaceutical, chemical and physical manipulation*

Pharmaceutical, chemical and physical manipulation is the use of substances and of methods which alter, attempt to alter or may reasonably be expected to alter the integrity and validity of urine samples used in doping controls, including, without limitation, catheterisation, urine substitution and or tampering, inhibition of renal excretion such as by probenecid and related compounds and alterations of testosterone and epitestosterone measurements such as epitestosterone* or bromantan administration.

* An epitestosterone concentration in the urine in excess of 200 nanograms per millilitre will have to be investigated by studies as in Article I.C (I).

The success or failure of the use of a prohibited substance or method is not material. It is sufficient that the said substance or procedure was used or attempted for the infraction to be considered as consummated.

III. Classes of drugs subject to certain restrictions

A. *Alcohol*

In agreement with the International Sports Federations and the responsible authorities, tests may be conducted for ethanol. The results may lead to sanctions.

B. *Marijuana*

In agreement with the International Sports Federations and the responsible authorities, tests may be conducted for cannabinoids (e.g. marijuana, hashish). The results may lead to sanctions.

C. *Local anaesthetics*

Injectable local anaesthetics are permitted under the following conditions:

a. bupivacaine, lidocaine, mepivacaine, procaine, etc. can be used but not cocaine. Vasoconstrictor agents (e.g. adrenaline) may be used in conjunction with local anaesthetics;

b. only local or intra-articular injections may be administered;

c. only when medically justified.

In agreement with International Sports Federations and the responsible authorities, notification of the permitted use may be necessary except for dental application. The details, including diagnosis, dose and route of administration, must be submitted prior to the competition or, if administered during the competition, immediately after injection, in writing to the relevant medical authority.

D. *Corticosteroids*

The use of corticosteroids is banned except:

a. for topical use (anal, aural, dermatological, nasal and ophthalmological) but not rectal;

b. by inhalation;

c. by intra-articular or local injection.

The IOC Medical Commission has introduced mandatory reporting of athletes requiring corticosteroids by inhalation for the treatment of asthma during competitions. Any team doctor wishing to administer corticosteroids by inhalation or by local or intra-articular injection to a competitor must give written notification prior to the competition to the relevant medical authority.

E. *Beta-blockers*

Some examples of beta-blockers are:

acebutolol, alprenolol, atenolol, labetalol, metoprolol, nadolol, oxprenolol, propranolol, sotalol

and related substances.

In agreement with the rules of the International Sports Federations, tests will be conducted in some sports, at the discretion of the responsible authorities. The results may lead to sanctions.

Summary of IOC regulations for drugs which need physician-written notification

Substances	Prohibited	Authorised with notification	Authorised without notification
Selected beta-agonists*	- Oral - Systemic injections	- Inhalatory	
Corticosteroids	- Oral - Systemic injections - Rectal	- Inhalatory - Local injections - Intra-articular injections	- Topical (anal, aural, dermatological, nasal, ophthalmological)
Local anaesthetics**	- Systemic injections		- Dental - Local injections*** - Intra-articular injections***

* salbutamol, salmeterol, terbutaline; all others beta-agonists are prohibited
** except cocaine, which is prohibited
*** in agreement with some International Sports Federations, notification may be necessary in some sports

Summary of urinary concentrations above which IOC-accredited laboratories must report findings for specific substances

cathine	> 5 micrograms / millilitre
ephedrine	> 5 micrograms / millilitre
epitestosterone	> 200 nanograms / millilitre
methylephedrine	> 5 micrograms / millilitre
morphine	> 1 microgram / millilitre
phenylpropanolamine	> 10 micrograms / millilitre
pseudoephedrine	> 10 micrograms / millilitre
T/E ratio	> 6

List of examples of prohibited substances

Caution

This is not an exhaustive list of prohibited substances. Many substances that do not appear on this list are prohibited under the term "and related substances".

All athletes are strongly advised only to take medicines which are prescribed by a medical doctor and to ensure that they contain only drugs that are not prohibited by the IOC Medical Commission or the responsible authorities.

Whenever an athlete is required to undergo a doping control it is essential that all medications and drugs taken or administered in the previous three days are declared on the doping control official record.

Stimulants

amineptine, amfepramone, amiphenazole, amphetamine, bambuterol, bromantan, caffeine, carphedon, cathine, cocaine, cropropamide, crotethamide, ephedrine, etamivan, etilamphetamine, etilefrine, fencamfamine, fenetylline, fenfluramine, formoterol, heptaminol, methylendioxyamphetamine, mefenorex, mephentermine, mesocarb, methamphetamine, methoxyphenamine, methylephedrine, methylphenidate, nikethamide, norfenfluramine, parahydroxyamphetamine, pemoline, pentylentetrazol, phendimetrazine, phentermine, phenylpropanolamine, pholedrine, pipradol, prolintane, propylhexedrine, pseudoephedrine, reproterol, salbutamol, salmeterol, selegiline, strychnine, terbutaline

Narcotics

dextromoramide, diamorphine (heroin), hydrocodone, methadone, morphine, pentazocine, pethidine

Anabolic agents

androstenedione, bambuterol, boldenone, clenbuterol, clostebol, danazol, dehydrochlormethyltestosterone, dehydroepiandrosterone (DHEA), dihydrotestosterone, drostanolone, fenoterol, formoterol, fluoxymesterone, formebolone, gestrinone, mesterolone, metandienone, metenolone, methandriol, methyltestosterone, mibolerone, nandrolone, norethandrolone, oxandrolone, oxymesterone, oxymetholone, reproterol, salbutamol, salmeterol, stanozolol, terbutaline, testosterone, trenbolone

Diuretics

acetazolamide, bendroflumethiazide, bumetanide, canrenone, chlortalidone, ethacrynic acid, furosemide, hydrochlorothiazide, indapamide, mannitol, mersalyl, spironolactone, triamterene

Masking agents

bromantan, epitestosterone, probenecid

Peptide hormones

ACTH, erythropoietin (EPO), hCG, hGH

Beta-blockers

acebutolol, alprenolol, atenolol, betaxolol, bisoprolol, bunolol, labetalol, metoprolol, nadodol, oxprenolol, propranolol, sotalol

Appendix B

Anti-doping Convention (ETS No. 135)

The member states of the Council of Europe, the other states party to the European Cultural Convention, and other states, signatory hereto,

Considering that the aim of the Council of Europe is to achieve a greater unity between its members for the purpose of safeguarding and realising the ideals and principles which are their common heritage and facilitating their economic and social progress;

Conscious that sport should play an important role in the protection of health, in moral and physical education and in promoting international understanding;

Concerned by the growing use of doping agents and methods by sportsmen and sportswomen throughout sport and the consequences thereof for the health of participants and the future of sport;

Mindful that this problem puts at risk the ethical principles and educational values embodied in the Olympic Charter, in the International Charter for Sport and Physical Education of Unesco and in Resolution (76) 41 of the Committee of Ministers of the Council of Europe, known as the "European Sport for All Charter";

Bearing in mind the anti-doping regulations, policies and declarations adopted by the international sports organisations;

Aware that public authorities and the voluntary sports organisations have complementary responsibilities to combat doping in sport, notably to ensure the proper conduct, on the basis of the principle of fair play, of sports events and to protect the health of those that take part in them;

Recognising that these authorities and organisations must work together for these purposes at all appropriate levels;

Recalling the resolutions on doping adopted by the Conference of European Ministers responsible for Sport, and in particular Resolution No. 1 adopted at the 6th Conference at Reykjavik in 1989;

Recalling that the Committee of Ministers of the Council of Europe has already adopted Resolution (67) 12 on the doping of athletes, Recommendation No. R (79) 8 on doping in sport, Recommendation No. R (84) 19 on the "European Anti-Doping Charter for Sport", and

Recommendation No. R (88) 12 on the institution of doping controls without warning outside competitions;

Recalling Recommendation No. 5 on doping adopted by the 2nd International Conference of Ministers and Senior Officials responsible for Sport and Physical Education organised by Unesco at Moscow (1988);

Determined however to take further and stronger co-operative action aimed at the reduction and eventual elimination of doping in sport using as a basis the ethical values and practical measures contained in those instruments,

Have agreed as follows:

Article 1 – Aim of the Convention

The Parties, with a view to the reduction and eventual elimination of doping in sport, undertake, within the limits of their respective constitutional provisions, to take the steps necessary to apply the provisions of this Convention.

Article 2 – Definition and scope of the Convention

1 For the purposes of this Convention:

   a "doping in sport" means the administration to sportsmen or sportswomen, or the use by them, of pharmacological classes of doping agents or doping methods;

   b "pharmacological classes of doping agents or doping methods" means, subject to paragraph 2 below, those classes of doping agents or doping methods banned by the relevant international sports organisations and appearing in lists that have been approved by the Monitoring Group under the terms of Article 11.1.b;

   c "sportsmen and sportswomen" means those persons who participate regularly in organised sports activities.

2 Until such time as a list of banned pharmacological classes of doping agents and doping methods is approved by the Monitoring Group under the terms of Article 11.1.b, the reference list in the appendix to this Convention shall apply.

Article 3 – Domestic co-ordination

1 The Parties shall co-ordinate the policies and actions of their government departments and other public agencies concerned with combating doping in sport.

2 They shall ensure that there is practical application of this Convention, and in particular that the requirements under Article 7 are met, by entrusting, where appropriate, the implementation of some of the provisions of this Convention to a designated governmental or non-governmental sports authority or to a sports organisation.

Article 4 – Measures to restrict the availability and use of banned doping agents and methods

1 The Parties shall adopt, where appropriate, legislation, regulations or administrative measures to restrict the availability (including provisions to control movement, possession, importation, distribution and sale) as well as the use in sport of banned doping agents and doping methods and in particular anabolic steroids.

2 To this end, the Parties or, where appropriate, the relevant non-governmental organisations shall make it a criterion for the grant of public subsidies to sports organisations that they effectively apply anti-doping regulations.

3 Furthermore, the Parties shall:

   a assist their sports organisations to finance doping controls and analyses, either by direct subsidies or grants, or by recognising the costs of such controls and analyses when determining the overall subsidies or grants to be awarded to those organisations;

   b take appropriate steps to withhold the grant of subsidies from public funds, for training purposes, to individual sportsmen and sportswomen who have been suspended following a doping offence in sport, during the period of their suspension;

   c encourage and, where appropriate, facilitate the carrying out by their sports organisations of the doping controls required by the competent international sports organisations whether during or outside competitions; and

   d encourage and facilitate the negotiation by sports organisations of agreements permitting their members to be tested by duly authorised doping control teams in other countries.

4 Parties reserve the right to adopt anti-doping regulations and to organise doping controls on their own initiative and on their own responsibility, provided that they are compatible with the relevant principles of this Convention.

Article 5 – Laboratories

1 Each Party undertakes:

   a either to establish or facilitate the establishment on its territory of one or more doping control laboratories suitable for consideration for accreditation under the criteria adopted by the relevant international sports organisations and approved by the Monitoring Group under the terms of Article 11.1.b;

   b or to assist its sports organisations to gain access to such a laboratory on the territory of another Party.

2 These laboratories shall be encouraged to:

  a take appropriate action to employ and retain, train and retrain qualified staff;

  b undertake appropriate programmes of research and development into doping agents and methods used, or thought to be used, for the purposes of doping in sport and into analytical biochemistry and pharmacology with a view to obtaining a better understanding of the effects of various substances upon the human body and their consequences for athletic performance;

  c publish and circulate promptly new data from their research.

Article 6 – Education

1 The Parties undertake to devise and implement, where appropriate in co-operation with the sports organisations concerned and the mass media, educational programmes and information campaigns emphasising the dangers to health inherent in doping and its harm to the ethical values of sport. Such programmes and campaigns shall be directed at both young people in schools and sports clubs and their parents, and at adult sportsmen and sportswomen, sports officials, coaches and trainers. For those involved in medicine, such educational programmes will emphasise respect for medical ethics.

2 The Parties undertake to encourage and promote research, in co-operation with the regional, national and international sports organisations concerned, into ways and means of devising scientifically-based physiological and psychological training programmes that respect the integrity of the human person.

Article 7 – Co-operation with sports organisations on measures to be taken by them

1 The Parties undertake to encourage their sports organisations and through them the international sports organisations to formulate and apply all appropriate measures, falling within their competence, against doping in sport.

2 To this end, they shall encourage their sports organisations to clarify and harmonise their respective rights, obligations and duties, in particular by harmonising their:

  a anti-doping regulations on the basis of the regulations agreed by the relevant international sports organisations;

  b lists of banned pharmacological classes of doping agents and banned doping methods, on the basis of the lists agreed by the relevant international sports organisations;

  c doping control procedures;

d disciplinary procedures, applying agreed international principles of natural justice and ensuring respect for the fundamental rights of suspected sportsmen and sportswomen ; these principles will include :

  i the reporting and disciplinary bodies to be distinct from one another ;

  ii the right of such persons to a fair hearing and to be assisted or represented ;

  iii clear and enforceable provisions for appealing against any judgement made ;

e procedures for the imposition of effective penalties for officials, doctors, veterinary doctors, coaches, physiotherapists and other officials or accessories associated with infringements of the anti-doping regulations by sportsmen and sportswomen ;

f procedures for the mutual recognition of suspensions and other penalties imposed by other sports organisations in the same or other countries.

3 Moreover, the Parties shall encourage their sports organisations :

a to introduce, on an effective scale, doping controls not only at, but also without advance warning at any appropriate time outside, competitions, such controls to be conducted in a way which is equitable for all sportsmen and sportswomen and which include testing and retesting of persons selected, where appropriate, on a random basis ;

b to negotiate agreements with sports organisations of other countries permitting a sportsman or sportswoman training in another country to be tested by a duly authorised doping control team of that country ;

c to clarify and harmonise regulations on eligibility to take part in sports events which will include anti-doping criteria ;

d to promote active participation by sportsmen and sportswomen themselves in the anti-doping work of international sports organisations ;

e to make full and efficient use of the facilities available for doping analysis at the laboratories provided for by Article 5, both during and outside sports competitions ;

f to study scientific training methods and to devise guidelines to protect sportsmen and sportswomen of all ages appropriate for each sport.

Article 8 – International co-operation

1 The Parties shall co-operate closely on the matters covered by this Convention and shall encourage similar co-operation amongst their sports organisations.

2 The Parties undertake :

a   to encourage their sports organisations to operate in a manner that promotes application of the provisions of this Convention within all the appropriate international sports organisations to which they are affiliated, including the refusal to ratify claims for world or regional records unless accompanied by an authenticated negative doping control report;

b   to promote co-operation between the staffs of their doping control laboratories established or operating in pursuance of Article 5;

c   to initiate bilateral and multilateral co-operation between their appropriate agencies, authorities and organisations in order to achieve, at the international level as well, the purposes set out in Article 4.1.

3   The Parties with laboratories established or operating in pursuance of Article 5 undertake to assist other Parties to enable them to acquire the experience, skills and techniques necessary to establish their own laboratories.

Article 9 – Provision of information

Each Party shall forward to the Secretary General of the Council of Europe, in one of the official languages of the Council of Europe, all relevant information concerning legislative and other measures taken by it for the purpose of complying with the terms of this Convention.

Article 10 – Monitoring Group

1   For the purposes of this Convention, a Monitoring Group is hereby set up.

2   Any Party may be represented on the Monitoring Group by one or more delegates. Each Party shall have one vote.

3   Any state mentioned in Article 14.1 which is not a Party to this Convention may be represented on the Monitoring Group by an observer.

4   The Monitoring Group may, by unanimous decision, invite any non-member state of the Council of Europe which is not a Party to the Convention and any sports or other professional organisation concerned to be represented by an observer at one or more of its meetings.

5   The Monitoring Group shall be convened by the Secretary General. Its first meeting shall be held as soon as reasonably practicable, and in any case within one year after the date of the entry into force of the Convention. It shall subsequently meet whenever necessary, on the initiative of the Secretary General or a Party.

6   A majority of the Parties shall constitute a quorum for holding a meeting of the Monitoring Group.

7   The Monitoring Group shall meet in private.

8   Subject to the provisions of this Convention, the Monitoring Group shall draw up and adopt by consensus its own Rules of Procedure.

Article 11

1   The Monitoring Group shall monitor the application of this Convention. It may in particular:

   a   keep under review the provisions of this Convention and examine any modifications necessary;

   b   approve the list, and any revision thereto, of pharmacological classes of doping agents and doping methods banned by the relevant international sports organisations, referred to in Articles 2.1 and 2.2, and the criteria for accreditation of laboratories, and any revision thereto, adopted by the said organisations, referred to in Article 5.1.a, and fix the date for the relevant decisions to enter into force;

   c   hold consultations with relevant sports organisations;

   d   make recommendations to the Parties concerning measures to be taken for the purposes of this Convention;

   e   recommend the appropriate measures to keep relevant international organisations and the public informed about the activities undertaken within the framework of this Convention;

   f   make recommendations to the Committee of Ministers concerning non-member states of the Council of Europe to be invited to accede to this Convention;

   g   make any proposal for improving the effectiveness of this Convention.

2   In order to discharge its functions, the Monitoring Group may, on its own initiative, arrange for meetings of groups of experts.

Article 12

After each meeting, the Monitoring Group shall forward to the Committee of Ministers of the Council of Europe a report on its work and on the functioning of the Convention.

Article 13 – Amendments to the articles of the Convention

1   Amendments to the articles of this Convention may be proposed by a party, the Committee of Ministers of the Council of Europe or the Monitoring Group.

2   Any proposal for amendment shall be communicated by the Secretary General of the Council of Europe to the states mentioned in Article 14 and to every state which has acceded to or has been invited to accede to this Convention in accordance with the provisions of Article 16.

3 Any amendment proposed by a Party or the Committee of Ministers shall be communicated to the Monitoring Group at least two months before the meeting at which it is to be considered. The Monitoring Group shall submit to the Committee of Ministers its opinion on the proposed amendment, where appropriate after consultation with the relevant sports organisations.

4 The Committee of Ministers shall consider the proposed amendment and any opinion submitted by the Monitoring Group and may adopt the amendment.

5 The text of any amendment adopted by the Committee of Ministers in accordance with paragraph 4 of this article shall be forwarded to the Parties for acceptance.

6 Any amendment adopted in accordance with paragraph 4 of this article shall come into force on the first day of the month following the expiration of a period of one month after all Parties have informed the Secretary General of their acceptance thereof.

Final clauses

Article 14

1 This Convention shall be open for signature by member states of the Council of Europe, other states party to the European Cultural Convention and non-member states which have participated in the elaboration of this Convention, which may express their consent to be bound by:

a signature without reservation as to ratification, acceptance or approval, or

b signature subject to ratification, acceptance or approval, followed by ratification, acceptance or approval.

2 Instruments of ratification, acceptance or approval shall be deposited with the Secretary General of the Council of Europe.

Article 15

1 The Convention shall enter into force on the first day of the month following the expiration of a period of one month after the date on which five states, including at least four member states of the Council of Europe, have expressed their consent to be bound by the Convention in accordance with the provisions of Article 14.

2 In respect of any signatory state which subsequently expresses its consent to be bound by it, the Convention shall enter into force on the first day of the month following the expiration of a period of one month after the date of signature or of the deposit of the instrument of ratification, acceptance or approval.

Article 16

1 After the entry into force of this Convention, the Committee of Ministers of the Council of Europe, after consulting the Parties, may invite to accede to the Convention any non-member State by a decision taken by the majority provided for in Article 20d of the Statute of the Council of Europe and by the unanimous vote of the representatives of the contracting states entitled to sit on the Committee.

2 In respect of any acceding state, the Convention shall enter into force on the first day of the month following the expiration of a period of one month after the date of the deposit of the instrument of accession with the Secretary General of the Council of Europe.

Article 17

1 Any state may, at the time of signature or when depositing its instrument of ratification, acceptance, approval or accession, specify the territory or territories to which this Convention shall apply.

2 Any state may, at any later date, by a declaration addressed to the Secretary General, extend the application of this Convention to any other territory specified in the declaration. In respect of such territory the Convention shall enter into force on the first day of the month following the expiration of a period of one month after the date of receipt of such declaration by the Secretary General.

3 Any declaration made under the two preceding paragraphs may, in respect of any territory mentioned in such declaration, be withdrawn by a notification addressed to the Secretary General. Such withdrawal shall become effective on the first day of the month following the expiration of a period of six months after the date of receipt of the notification by the Secretary General.

Article 18

1 Any Party may, at any time, denounce this Convention by means of a notification addressed to the Secretary General of the Council of Europe.

2 Such denunciation shall become effective on the first day of the month following the expiration of a period of six months after the date of receipt of the notification by the Secretary General.

Article 19

The Secretary General of the Council of Europe shall notify the Parties, the other member states of the Council of Europe, the other States party to the European Cultural Convention, the non-member states which have participated in the elaboration of this Convention and any state which has acceded or has been invited to accede to it of:

a any signature in accordance with Article 14;

b the deposit of any instrument of ratification, acceptance, approval or accession in accordance with Article 14 or 16;

c any date of entry into force of this Convention in accordance with Articles 15 and 16;

d any information forwarded under the provisions of Article 9;

e any report prepared in pursuance of the provisions of Article 12;

f any proposal for amendment or any amendment adopted in accordance with Article 13 and the date on which the amendment comes into force;

g any declaration made under the provisions of Article 17;

h any notification made under the provisions of Article 18 and the date on which the denunciation takes effect;

i any other act, notification or communication relating to this Convention.

In witness whereof the undersigned, being duly authorised thereto, have signed this Convention.

Done at Strasbourg, the 16th day of November 1989, in English and French, both texts being equally authentic, in a single copy which shall be deposited in the archives of the Council of Europe. The Secretary General of the Council of Europe shall transmit certified copies to each member state of the Council of Europe, to the other States party to the European Cultural Convention, to the non-member states which have participated in the elaboration of this Convention and to any state invited to accede to it.

Appendix

List of prohibited classes of substances and prohibited methods[1]

---

1. For the latest list of substances prohibited by the International Olympic Committee, adopted by the Monitoring Group on the Anti-doping Convention in March 1998, see Appendix A.

Appendix C

Chart of signatures and ratifications to the Anti-doping Convention (ETS No. 135)

Last up-date: 28 October 1998

Opening for signature   Place: Strasbourg   Date: 16 November 1989

Entry into force: Conditions: five ratifications including four member states

Date: 1 March 1990

Member states	Date of signature	Date of ratification or accession	Date of entry into force	R: Reservations D: Declarations T: Territorial Decl.
Albania	02/02/95			
Andorra				
Austria	10/05/90	10/07/91	01/09/91	
Belgium	16/11/89			
Bulgaria	24/03/92	01/06/92	01/08/92	
Croatia	Accession	27/01/93	01/03/93	
Cyprus	20/06/91	02/02/94	01/04/94	
Czech Rep.	28/04/95 (1)	28/04/95 (1)	01/06/95	
Denmark	16/11/89 (1)	16/11/89 (1)	01/03/90	T
Estonia	14/05/93	20/11/97	01/01/98	
Finland	16/11/89	26/04/90	01/06/90	
France	16/11/89	21/01/91	01/03/91	T
Germany	27/05/92	28/04/94	01/06/94	
Greece	10/10/90	06/03/96	01/05/96	
Hungary	29/01/90 (1)	29/01/90 (1)	01/03/90	
Iceland	25/03/91 (1)	25/03/91 (1)	01/05/91	
Ireland	25/06/92			
Italy	16/11/89	12/02/96	01/04/96	
Latvia	23/01/97	23/01/97	01/03/97	
Liechtenstein	16/11/89			
Lithuania	01/04/93	17/05/96	01/07/96	
Luxembourg	16/11/89	21/06/96	01/08/96	
Malta	09/09/94			
Moldova				
Netherlands	04/12/90	11/04/95	01/06/95	T
Norway	16/11/89 (1)	16/11/89 (1)	01/03/90	
Poland	16/11/89	07/09/90	01/11/90	
Portugal	14/06/90	17/03/94	01/05/94	
Romania	16/06/94			

Member states	Date of signature	Date of ratification or accession	Date of entry into force	R: Reservations D: Declarations T: Territorial Decl.
Russia	Accession	12/02/91	01/04/91	
San Marino	16/11/89	31/01/90	01/03/90	
Slovak Rep.	06/05/93¹	06/05/93¹	01/07/93	
Slovenia	Accession	02/07/92	01/09/92	
Spain	16/11/89	20/05/92	01/07/92	
Sweden	16/11/89	29/06/90	01/08/90	
Switzerland	16/11/89	05/11/92	01/01/93	
"the former Yugoslav Republic of Macedonia"	Accession	30/03/94	01/05/94	
Turkey	16/11/89	22/11/93	01/01/94	
Ukraine	02/07/98			
United Kingdom	16/11/89 (1)	16/11/89 (1)	01/03/90	T
Non member states	Date of signature	Date of ratification or accession	Date of entry into force	R: Reservations D: Declarations T: Territorial Decl.
Armenia				
Australia	Accession	5/10/94	01/12/94	
Azerbaijan				
Belarus				
Bosnia and Herzegovina	Accession	29/12/94	01/02/95	
Canada	6/03/96 (1)	06/03/96 (1)	01/05/96	
Georgia				
Holy See				
Monaco				
United States				

* Treaty open for signature by the member states, the other states party to the European Cultural Convention and non-member states which have participated in its elaboration, and for accession by other non-member states.

1. Signature without reservation as to ratification.